I Die, But My
Memory Lives On

Henning Mankell

TRANSLATED FROM THE SWEDISH BY
LAURIE THOMPSON

NEW YORK · LONDON

The New Press gratefully acknowledges Pathfinder International for granting permission to reprint Peter Kanyi's memory book in I Die, But My Memory Lives On. Since 1957, Pathfinder International has supported high-quality family planning and reproductive health services that improve the lives of women, men, and children throughout the developing world. Pathfinder's work in Kenya is made possible through the generous support of the U. S. Agency for International Development. We also wish to recognize the work of the Kenya Network of Women Living with AIDS (KENWA), a local group that encourages parents living with HIV/AIDS to create these important documents for their children. Working in over twenty countries throughout Africa, Latin America, Asia, and the Near East, Pathfinder is committed to making family planning and reproductive health services available to all who want them. For further information, please visit **www.pathfinder.org**.

Requests for permission to reproduce selections
from this book should be mailed to:
Permissions Department, The New Press,
38 Greene Street, New York, NY 10013.

Originally published as *Jag dör, men minnet lever*
by Leopard Förlag, Stockholm, 2003
English translation first published in Great Britain
by The Harvill Press, London, 2004
Published in the United States by The New Press, New York, 2005
Distributed by W. W. Norton & Company, Inc., New York

ISBN 1-59558-013-1 (hc.)
CIP data available

The New Press was established in 1990 as a not-for-profit alternative
to the large, commercial publishing houses currently dominating the
book publishing industry. The New Press operates in the public interest rather than for private gain, and is committed to publishing, in
innovative ways, works of educational, cultural, and community value
that are often deemed insufficiently profitable.

www.thenewpress.com

Book design and composition by Kelly Too
This book was set in Berling

Printed in the United States of America
2 4 6 8 10 9 7 5 3 1

I Die, But My Memory Lives On

ALSO BY HENNING MANKELL

Faceless Killers
The Dogs of Riga
The White Lioness
Sidetracked
The Fifth Woman
One Step Behind
Firewall
The Return of the Dancing Master
Before the Frost

Contents

Foreword by Archbishop Desmond Tutu
vii

The Mango Plant
2

Afterword by Samuel A. Worthington
107

Foreword

by Archbishop Desmond Tutu

Henning Mankell is a most remarkable man. The bestselling author of detective stories in many countries, he has become almost a cult figure in much of the world (though perhaps it is his great creation, chief inspector Kurt Wallander of the Ystad provincial police force, who's really the cult figure).

A talented artist who with strokes of his brush evokes the dampness and cold of Sweden and also the smoke-filled atmosphere of the desert townships in South Africa, Henning Mankell keeps us filled with anticipation. And as we follow with bated breath Kurt's intuition, stalking his prey, we wonder all the while whether the underworld will get the best of our hero. And we all sigh with deep relief when the criminal is cornered and good triumphs, as we hoped it would, over evil.

It is one thing to consider the creator of Kurt Wallander, but every bit as interesting and important are Henning Mankell's remarkable efforts to build bridges between Africa and Europe, efforts begun at an early age, with the hope of bringing education and reconciliation between these two continents. These were the efforts for which Mankell was honored with the Tolerance Prize in Germany in the Spring of 2004.

Henning Mankell has dedicated himself to the fight against AIDS, which is devastating the African continent and sub-continent. Thank to his efforts, memory books and Project AIDS have done an enormous amount to raise awareness of the epidemic. By encouraging parents to recall their life stories, not just for their children, but also for humanity, Henning Mankell has given a great gift to the world. Through South Africa's Truth and Reconciliation Commission I have been amazed at how important telling one's stories turned out to be in helping people to heal. Their enormous therapeutic value cannot be overestimated. A young man who had been blinded by police action in his township came to the commission and told his story, and he was asked afterwards, "How do you feel? You are still blind." He replied, "Ah yes, but now I can see."

Henning Mankell has used his considerable talents as an artist to build bridges, much as Daniel Barenboim, the previous prize winner, has used his music to advance the course of peace in the Middle East. Through his works, Henning Mankell has expressed his belief in solidarity between different peoples. I, as a Christian, have been trying to do much the same kind of thing. God's dream is that we realize that we are all God's children, that we are members of one family: God's family, a family, in which there are no outsiders, only insiders—all belong. All are held in the embrace of a love that will not let go. Every one of us is precious. White, black, rich, or poor. All. Gay. Lesbian. All belong in this family. God has no enemies. So that a Bush, a Bin Laden, a Saddam Hussein, an Arafat, a Sharon, all, all belong.

Henning Mankell was born on February 3, 1948, in what he has described as a damp, cold part of Sweden. Together with his brother and sister, he was raised by a divorced father, a judge, who was so caring that Henning did not miss his mother. At thirteen, he went to Stockholm and worked in a theater. And he fulfilled his childhood dream when, in 1972, he went to Africa for the first time. As he said, much later, Africa made him a better European, and gave him perspective.

Since 1985, Henning Mankell has commuted between Sweden and Maputo, Mozambique. He writes with a rhythm, devoting mornings to writing so that in the afternoon he can be involved with his beloved theater company. When the country was devastated by floods in 2000 and hundreds of people were dying, Henning Mankell provided assistance together with Doctors Without Borders, lamenting the fact that Western aid had come too late and was too little.

Mankell has also written a play called *Butterfly Blues* for a theater in Graz, Austria, the land of Joerg Haider, famous for his racist anti-immigration policies. The play is about daily discrimination and harassment of the so-called Third World immigrants. Some of the actors in the play came from Mozambique and others from Austria, and they did not understand one another's languages. Henning Mankell's vision is of human beings from different origins and places living together, not separated by the walls, stones, wars, or laws which divide them.

Henning Mankell uses a range of different literary genres—mysteries, novels, stories about teenagers. He says that his crime stories are merely mirrors held up to examine society. He asks the question, Should a society be based on solidarity or not? And there is no doubt about what his answer is. Henning Mankell has had the courage and the passion to challenge the affluent First World not to be so obsessed with their own issues such as capitalism, alienation, and political disillusionment. He challenges the citizens of that part of God's world to be concerned about poverty, about hunger, about violence, which don't happen exclusively in the so-called Third World.

· · ·

We are all in the world bound up in a common humanity. A person is a person through other persons. I can be human only in relationships. I can be me only when you are you. We are bound up in a common humanity that shares the vulnerability of being human, but also shares the strengths of solidarity.

The world is much more insecure now than it has ever been. Military might does not mean security. The war against terror can never be won, so long as conditions exist which make people so desperate that they resort to acts of desperation. We belong together. We can be human only together. We can survive only together. We can be free only together.

When we hear a cry for help on the stairs, we can either turn on our televisions louder or we can help. Henning Mankell would rather fall over dead than turn on his television louder. And he shows us that we do have a choice. As Martin Luther King Jr. once said, either we learn to live together as brothers (and sisters) or we perish together as fools.

Henning Mankell shares with Kurt Wallander the love of music, and of Mozart. But most importantly, he shares with him a belief in the counsel contained in "Proverbs" to speak up. We must speak for those who cannot speak for themselves. *I Die, But My Memory Lives On* is a deeply moving account of Henning Mankell's personal responses to AIDS and its victims, both parents and the children left behind far too soon. In the midst of the death and suffering, a young girl plants a tree. She nurtures it as a fragment of life that will grow and survive and, like the memory books, outlive this global crisis. By highlighting and humanizing this catastrophe, Henning Mankell shows a way to help. As Mankell writes in *I Die, But My Memory Lives On*, "These memory books, small exercise books with pasted-in pictures and texts . . . could prove to be the most important documents our time has produced."

I Die, But My Memory Lives On

A MEMORY BOOK

Dedicated to PETER with love
It's My Life—You Are My Child

I Was Born In . . .

*I was born on Tuesday August 16th 1965 at Nyen
General Hospital in the village of Kihuyo. My mother
had a difficult time when I was born. Although she
had only just married, my father abandoned her.
The hospital would not let my mother take me home
because she could not afford to pay the doctor's bill.
She went to ask my grandmother for the money but
didn't get it. As I write this, remembering how my
Mom was treated at this time is very painful to me.*

The Mango Plant

· 1 ·

It has been two weeks since I met Aida in her village, a few miles north of Kampala in Uganda. The earth there was red and the banana trees grew in dense clumps. It has been two weeks since she showed me where she had hidden her mango plant.

· 2 ·

I had gone to Kampala by car from the airport in Entebbe. Kampala is a cluster of hills, seven or eight, and tucked tightly between these hills, dotted by elegant houses with large gardens, was the town itself, with far too much traffic, far too many people.

I was brought up in the Reserve not in town. When I was young I filled my days fetching water—the nearest source was some three kilometers away, collecting firewood in the forest, chasing wild animals (though we were careful never to go near lions) and helping my grandmother with cooking. We also played games—Tappo was a game where you hid until tapped on the shoulder at which point you had to go to find other people to tap. I also liked to run long distance races and attend music festivals.

Africa is always a conflict of opposites, of urban chaos and vast, empty regions.

I say Africa, but Africa can be divided into any number of parts. Some countries within this continent are the size of all of western Europe. There is no clear-cut, single entity that you can think of as Africa. This continent has many faces, but wherever I have been the dense urban chaos and vast, empty spaces have always been side by side.

Aida's village is like all the other African villages I know. The houses are made of clay or sheets of corrugated iron or the strangest mixture of materials that happened to be at hand for the builders. But all of the lived-in houses I saw in her village had roofs.

On the other hand, there were also abandoned houses that had collapsed. When I asked why this had happened, I was told that the people who had lived there had died of AIDS.

African houses often have a distinctive character. Perhaps you could say it is the equivalent of the Scandinavian passion for ornate carpentry at the end of the nineteenth century. In Aida's village, two doors from an old American car make up the gate in a ramshackle fence around a house where a hairdresser plies his trade. As we pass, he is cutting a customer's hair in the shade of a tree. Shortly before we came to Aida's house—or rather her mother, Christine's, house—I notice two men, their backs running with sweat, building a wall between two corner posts with rusty pieces from old oil drums.

African houses in rural areas are a hymn to the imagination, if you like. But of course they are also an expression of poverty and destitution. Around the houses are small gardens, gravel roads meandering all over the place, and apologies for fences. Nearly all of the windows have broken panes with curtains flapping behind them.

Life proceeds at a leisurely pace in these villages. Haste is a human error that has not established very deep roots in the African countryside.

· 3 ·

But none of this is important. I do not need to describe houses and roads, as if this were some sort of travelogue from a country in Africa. I have other reasons for being here.

In this very village, Aida's village, there is something else that all the other villages in the area have in common. Many of the villagers have AIDS. Many are already dead from the disease. You can already see the big gap: lots of children, quite a few old people, but not many in between. AIDS generally kills people from fifteen to twenty years old to those in their early fifties. The old people have to look after their grandchildren when the children's parents die. When the old people die, the children are left to look after themselves. What that means is obvious to everybody. Children who have to be one another's parents have a pretty distorted start in life. They slip up.

Even if life goes on as usual, it is as if there is an endless silence all around them. Daily events, everyday events, take place under a cold shadow. Many people, too many people, are going to die. That shadow is not black, nor is it white. It is just not visible. It is like a cold gust of wind.

In Aida's village the silence was so tangible that it did not need to be visible.

· 4 ·

There were various sorts of waiting among the people I met in Uganda. Those who knew they were infected and spent every day looking for symptoms. Those who didn't know, those who had refused to be tested, but nevertheless looked for symptoms every day, from the moment they opened their eyes.

But there is another kind of waiting. For the people who find themselves in the same position as Aida. She is only a child, she knows that she is not infected, but she will become mother to herself and her siblings the moment that responsibility is passed on to her.

Our Family Came From . . .

*Our family, which is known as Mbari ya Wangombe,
came from a village called Kihuyo in the Nyen
District of central Kenya. You should be aware that
you come from a well-known family. Wangombe is a
prestigious name because my great grandfather was a
wealthy chieftain and a prominent anti-colonialist.
Family legend recounts that on a raid of a Masai
mauyato he stole some cattle and also a baby girl.
He gave the girl to his eldest wife who brought her
up. When she was older, Wangombe took the girl as
his wife. She then gave birth to Ruga, who was my
grandfather, and he married Wambui who I am
named after. My grandmother had no record of
the precise year when she was born. In those days
people marked their birth dates by referring to some
important event such as a drought, a locust invasion,
or a famine. Times were hard then. My grandmother
lost 6 children because there were no hospitals. One
of her children was Wagura (Kariuki). That's who
you're named after. That is our origin.*

*Unfortunately your grandfather died just one year
before you were born so you never met him. My
father was a man of his word and the envy of my
heart. He was born in 1939. He was a spirited,*

And now I see her in a dream. It has not been very long since we were together. The last I remember of her, she was waving vigorously. Even when she could no longer see me nor the car, no doubt she went on waving.

We all do that when we hope against hope that somebody will change their mind, decide to do something different. Come back, break off the journey, stay behind.

· 5 ·

But in the dream she's dead. Her face appears as an unfinished wooden sculpture. That upsets me. And it's not right. It must be somebody else, somebody who looks like her. She is not the one who is dead. It is others who are dying. Not Aida. She is alive. She hasn't grown thinner, she isn't covered in sores, she hasn't lost all her strength so that all she can do is lie on a bast mat in the shade, staring up at the sky or at the big leaves of the banana trees.

· 6 ·

The answer is obvious, of course. I'm mixing things up. Dreams do mix things up. The first thing that strikes me when I meet Aida is how much she *independent-minded man. Sometimes, after he had been drinking, he would get into fights with his employer and then the family would have to pack up and leave the plantation where he was working. As a result we moved around a lot and, as a child, I couldn't even imagine what it would be like to stay in one place for any length of time.*

But there was also a positive side to my father. He loved me and me alone. Though he fought with other members of our family, beating them and banishing them, he never did this to me. We were very close. I was the first born and had to take responsibility for my younger brothers and sisters. It was not an easy task and even today this burden still rests on my shoulders. At home, I became Dad's watchdog, reporting gossip and misconduct to him. My brothers and sisters didn't like this and when he was away I would be severely reprimanded for the simplest of mistakes. In order to avoid this I would often accompany Dad when he went out drinking. This only served to unify still further his heart with mine.

When my Dad died I thought the world had come to an end. For the first time I felt all things must cease but, no, the sun still set

looks like her mother. And Christine, her mother, is ill. She may well be dead by now. The same applies to Aida's aunt. Both of them could well be dead, even though it has only been a couple of weeks since I was talking to them.

Aida's face is there, out in the mist. She comes very close to me.

· 7 ·

One windy day, in the middle of this most unstable June, just before I start to write down my story about Aida, her mango plant, and all the people around her in Uganda waiting to die of AIDS, I visit one of the many medieval churches on the island of Gotland. It doesn't matter which one. The darkness of these old stone-built churches is the breath they all breathe. Darkness has no individual identity. Darkness is eternal, and has no face, no name.

A lone man is tending a grave. The gate at the churchyard entrance is black and heavy. The handle is difficult to turn.

Somebody, a friend from the old days, once told me that dark churches made him afraid of death. It is precisely the opposite for me. In the darkness of a medieval church on Gotland, time ceases to exist. Or perhaps all time, the past, the present, the future—all of them are compressed into a shared moment. Going into certain churches you feel at *that day, cows came home and were milked, supper was cooked and people went to sleep at night. In other words, life continued. But, for me, nothing was ever the same again.*

I remember another family member telling me during Dad's burial "Cry as much as you want because he's dead and dead completely, but you, you must live." She told me "As long as it's not you who is dead, life continues and even when you die, life will continue for others." At the time I hated to hear this but now I realize the importance of her words and what they imply. I have learned quite a number of things. As long as you are alive, no matter what happens, be it having HIV infection, or AIDS, or being nothing at all, life must continue.

peace the moment the door closes behind you. Nothing else is needed. The church creates its own universe.

· 8 ·

I have a special reason for coming to this particular church. It feels cool within these thick stone walls. The noise of the lawnmower working away outside cannot penetrate the stone or the windows.

I contemplate the frescoes on one of the walls. The skeleton of Death is chasing a human being, smiling wryly and wielding his scythe. The man is terrified of Death, whose arrival is always untimely. In this ancient place I am faced with pictures of the Black Death, the Plague. Time stands still, but the reality of past time is present even so.

It occurs to me that, among all these images of Gotland peasants, I can see Aida. A black face among the medieval farmers from Tingstäde and Roma. Solidarity among men and women is as much present in horror as it is in joy.

Among the people portrayed are her mother, her brothers, and her sisters. Death pursues them all through the ages. The images frozen onto the walls of the medieval church are in some ways a moving picture. The figures come running towards me, gliding through arrested time.

Then it was the Plague, now it is AIDS. Then it

was bacteria, now it is a virus. But death is never visible. Where does the illness come from? Where do the sores come from, what causes the emaciation?

Why should bacteria and viruses be so small that they cannot be seen? Why should they have this unfair advantage?

· 9 ·

I sit in a pew in the dark interior and reflect. When did I first hear about this insidious and mysterious illness that seemed at first only to affect gay men on the west coast of America?

I cannot remember.

I have searched my memory and gone through newspapers from the early 1980s to see if there might be a headline I recognize, that could help me fix on a specific date. At certain times in my life I have kept detailed and seriously intended diaries, but they have not been able to help me either. I cannot find a moment that I can point to with any degree of certainty and say: this is when I realized that something momentous was happening. A new epidemic illness had put mankind under threat. Nor do I recall any conversations with friends about the illness, definitely not before 1985 or 1986.

Perhaps it was the sight of the actor Rock Hudson on a stretcher in Paris. I remember that distinctly. There were photographs on the front pages of all the big newspapers. It was immediately clear that the man who—most notably with Doris Day—had made so many films over so many years in which he had played a husband in an idealized and hence dishonest American marriage was in fact homosexual. What had he been thinking of as he wandered around in his striped pajamas, always immaculately ironed, Doris Day at his side, also smiling nonstop and fussing around?

Now he was dying, not at all old. His last journey to Paris in a chartered airplane was reminiscent of the handicapped faithful who tried to recover their health by going on a pilgrimage to a shrine of the Madonna. A last desperate attempt to keep death at bay by trying a new form of treatment that was said to be available in France.

I remember reading that he slept twenty-three hours a day. The one hour he was awake he devoted to telling stories about his life. I shuddered.

That news photograph of Rock Hudson is among my earliest intimations of AIDS. At that time we had not yet been exposed to the mass of pictures and documentation. All the photographs from Africa of anonymous men and women, emaciated bodies, sunken eyes, people without hope, without strength.

I also recall a young African quoted in a newspaper: "Must we die because we are in love?"

But the first decisive impression? I am pretty sure it was Rock Hudson. It was as if a sculpture guaranteed unbreakable had nevertheless shattered. And yet I am not absolutely sure.

On the other hand, I can say precisely when AIDS became real for me, when I myself became frightened of the illness, terrified that I had been infected.

I knew, of course, how one became infected. And, yes, I had friends who were doctors and they assured me that there were no shortcuts that the infection could take to attack me. Nevertheless, the fear was there. I know it is a fear that I shared and still share with many people.

· 10 ·

It is easy to lie about this. Easy to boast that one has never experienced any trace of the irrational fear of being infected, despite the fact that common sense tells you that you have not been exposed to any risks. That is how it has always been. People ten or so years older than I am have stories to tell about a similarly needless fear of being stricken with syphilis. They will tell you about the Wasserman test they had to take before being accepted as a blood donor, and that it was a good way of establishing that one did not in fact have a syphilis bomb ticking away in one's body. As a teenager I remember being scared stiff by stories about gonorrhea. I don't think I've spoken about venereal disease with a single person who hasn't felt a cold shiver run down his spine at least once in his life.

But the fear of HIV and AIDS? I recall it very clearly. There was a period in the 1980s when the fear was especially widespread. All kinds of horror stories were circulating in the mass media. There was an account of how a passenger suffering from AIDS was not allowed to board an American flight from China. The captain refused to allow him on board. There were those who argued that people infected should be branded, or tattooed on the groin. Or why not herd them together and maroon them on remote islands to await their deaths?

There are moments when the frescoes in the Gotland churches seem to be speaking directly to us, right now. Not only addressing us, but speaking about us, and that we are part of their story.

It was also in the mid-1980s that people started looking for scapegoats. Politicians with extreme views started fishing in muddy waters, but they were not the only ones looking for scapegoats; a lot of "ordinary" people were also carried away by the fear. Homosexuals were branded the guilty party, the ones who were spreading the disease. Just as in the past it was the Jews who had been blamed for spreading the deadly plague by infecting people's wells.

When I Was Growing Up, This Is What It Was Like . . .

Life was not as comfortable as it is today. That's why I try to offer you the best that I can so that you don't experience what I had to go through when growing up. We lived on coffee plantations and picked coffee to earn our living. Even when I was quite young I had to pick coffee to boost my parent's daily income— I thought all people earned their living through coffee picking.

In those days wearing shoes was unheard of. I wore my first pair of shoes when I was in class 6. Believe me, I could not tell the difference between the left and right shoe. The fact that our family came from a poor background meant that we couldn't have more than one dress. I could only get a new dress when the one I was wearing was so worn out that it couldn't be patched any more.

In 1972, my Mother formally separated from my Dad and I was left under his care until 1975. For these years I was unable to attend school and didn't return to education until Mom and Dad got back together again. During this period I was taken to stay with my grandma but she was not happy to have me there and did all she could to frustrate and discourage us from

So it was the homosexuals who should all be branded, especially if they were black men. All black men seeking asylum in Europe should be subjected to HIV tests. Those who were infected should be turned away.

When the history of AIDS in the 1980s comes to be written, a lot of ugly truths will emerge with full and frightening force.

In our part of the world, at least the absolute terror is no longer with us. There are nevertheless some people still who maintain that the AIDS epidemic is the wages of sin. The scapegoats exist, be they asylum seekers, homosexual men, or Russian prostitutes.

·11·

I remember well the moment when I myself was struck by this fear. It was in Lusaka, in November 1987. I was staying at the Ridgeway Hotel. I'd just driven there from Kabompo, where I was living at the time, high up toward Zambia's northwestern border with Angola. I was on my way to Europe. The flight was going to leave the following day. I was dirty and tired after the long journey and had checked into the Ridgeway. That evening, after dinner, I went for a walk around the hotel and its grounds. At one end of the hotel I discovered the entrance to a casino. I took a look inside the dimly *staying. I remember days when we didn't have enough to eat. I had to work very hard, looking after cattle, fetching water and firewood, and cooking. I longed to be reunited with my parents, something I don't think they appreciated. Despite all this, I excelled at school when I returned there, passing exams with flying colors. I especially liked math, biology, and chemistry.*

lit room and was immediately solicited by several prostitutes who were stationed along the wall next to the roulette table. Young and pretty. Dangerous. I thought at once that several of them were bound to be infected. How many men in my situation, visitors to the hotel or the casino, would succumb to the temptation offered by the girls? A night in the hotel, then good-bye. But death would be there already, inside their skin, sowed into their blood, flowing through their veins.

I drew back in alarm. There before me, a smiling mask, was death. The virus I was so afraid of. The girls were indeed young and pretty, but what they were offering me was death. I would have to be an idiot to accept. And, what is more, be willing to pay for it.

The fear, irrational though it was, stayed with me for many years, certainly until the mid-1990s. Perhaps it is still there, even if my fits of baseless anxiety have become increasingly rare. I took a test once, even though I had absolutely no reason to be scared. But scared I was, no matter what. And, I know, many others, very many, have experienced that same fear.

· 12 ·

It was in Zambia too that I first encountered someone who quite definitely did have AIDS. It was a young man. He staggered off an overcrowded bus in Kabompo. He fell at the feet of the people who had come to meet him. He was taken to the hospital in a wheelbarrow. He was as thin as it is possible to be.

Two days later he was dead. He had only just made it home from Kitwe, back to his mother in order to die close to her. His name was Richard. He was seventeen, and he was not gay. This was in 1988.

·13·

At the same place, Kabompo, I listened to a Dutch doctor giving a talk about this terrifying disease. It was an evening during the rainy season. The roads were a sea of mud, but people came from all points of the compass, and a number of tribal chieftains were there. The premises belonged to one of the missionary groups and were the biggest in Kabompo but still the place was packed to the rafters. There were others standing outside, looking in through the open windows. It was unbearably hot.

The doctor described in simple, straightforward terms—and what he said was translated into the local language by an interpreter—what happened in the body once HIV had entered the blood. He said that promiscuity was the principal culprit in the spread of the disease, and there was a rising hum, like a swarm of bees, from the women present. It was a pregnant moment. When the doctor had finished, one of the chieftains, a very old man, rose to his feet. He said: "We must all protect ourselves. For the sake of our children. There must be a stop to all unnecessary travelling. Families must stick together. Men must remain faithful to their women, women to their men. If not, we shall all die."

That was in 1988, during the rainy season. I often wonder how many of those who were there listening to the Dutch doctor were already infected. And how many of them are still alive today.

·14·

The mist is dispersing. I stare out to sea and I think about Aida and her mango plant. When she showed it to me, I felt no doubt that it was one of the moments I would remember for as long as I live.

·15·

Just how it came about, I don't know. Nor do I know when Aida made up her mind to take me into her confidence and share her secret with me. But I saw the plant the second time I visited her and her family.

The first time I met her, it was a very hot day.

We left Kampala early so as to avoid being stuck in the chaotic traffic that envelops the city's roads every morning. Beatrice, who was the person helping me make contact with people carrying the disease and writing memory books, had told Christine that I would be coming. At that time I didn't know Christine had a daughter called Aida. In fact, I knew only two things about Christine: that she had AIDS, and that she was prepared to talk to me about it.

When we left Kampala that morning I felt the same distaste I'd been feeling ever since arriving in Uganda. There was something almost obscene about asking fatally ill people to talk about their suffering and their fate with a complete stranger. Somebody who, to make matters worse, had flown in from a distant corner of the world—Europe, the West—in which the terrible disease had almost been tamed and turned into a chronic but not necessarily fatal disease. The same disease that now is killing indiscriminately the length and breadth of the African continent and in other parts of the Third World.

I had slept badly because I had been worrying about the task ahead. My unease was not difficult to understand. I was dreading it because I knew I would find the fate of Christine and the rest of them very hard to take.

Beatrice had given us very efficient directions how to get there. We turned off the main road and,

as always in Africa, we immediately found ourselves deep in a different world, a world usually,
but wrongly, called the real Africa. Africa is always
"real," whether it be savannah or slum, old ramshackle urban district or a grim and difficult-to-
pin-down shadowland between bush and desert.

Christine had two houses. In one of them lived
her mother and father and some of her brothers
and sisters. When I arrived and got out of the car,
the first thing I saw was her father, who was sitting
peeling some kind of vegetable I had never seen
before. He was unshaven but very dignified.
Eventually I discovered that he was about eighty,
although nobody could be sure exactly how old.
He had a keen eye, and was surrounded by an
aura that immediately captivated anyone who
approached him.

He went on peeling his vegetables all the time I
was talking to Christine. Occasionally some child
or perhaps his wife or one of the other women
would give him something to drink.

He was like a measurer of time who would
reject a normal clock with scorn. For him, a better
way of measuring progress in his life and that of
others was peeling vegetables.

Christine was thin and tired. I could see at once
that she had made an effort to look her best for our
meeting. Her choice of clothes, her face carefully
made-up, her meticulously brushed hair. She was
typical of all the people suffering from AIDS

whom I met during my visit to Uganda: the last thing they would be forced to surrender was their dignity. That was the ditch that had to be defended at all costs: after that there was nothing but death, and it often struck quickly once their dignity had been lost.

Christine said: "I have a daughter."

We were sitting on two brown stools behind the open but covered room that the family used to prepare food. Christine said something in her native tongue. Her daughter emerged from a clump of banana trees. She was wearing a dark blue skirt, which was ragged and torn, and a red blouse, and she was bare-footed. She was slim and tall and took after her mother: they had the same features around their mouths and noses and eyes. Aida was shy; she spoke in a low voice and her eyes were cast down. When I shook her hand, she withdrew it as quickly as she could.

Aida was nowhere to be seen for the rest of my long conversation with her mother. It was almost afternoon, when we had to leave to drive back to Kampala and had other appointments, before I saw Aida again. She was with Christine's mother and some of the other girls, not Christine's daughters but the daughters of her sister. One sister had already died of AIDS. They were preparing dinner. I watched Aida fetch the vegetables that Christine's father had been peeling all day.

Christine said: "When I'm gone, Aida will have

to take on a lot of responsibility. I am trying to live for as long as I can for her sake."

"Does she know about it?"

Christine looked at me in surprise.

"Of course she knows about it."

"What did you tell her?"

"What had to be said. She will become the mother of her brothers and sisters, and if my parents are still alive she will become their new daughter once I'm gone."

"How did she react?"

"She was distressed. What else would you expect?"

We went to the car, which was parked in the shade of some tall trees whose name I have never managed to remember. I had said good-bye to everybody, and figured out that Christine's family comprised sixteen people. Christine, who had been a schoolteacher and still worked whenever she had the strength, was the only one in this large family who had any income, and even that was extremely modest. She had a very direct way of assessing her wages in relation to her own fate.

"The monthly cost of antiretroviral drugs is precisely twice what I earn."

She shook her head before continuing.

"Obviously, you have to ask yourself if it is the drugs that are too expensive, or if it's me who isn't earning enough. The answer is straightforward. My small wage has always been sufficient to feed my

Your Father . . .

Your father was born in a place called Limura. His full name was Joseph Kamau Kanuk. When I first met him in 1988 we fell for each other straight away. We went to the same medical school. He later qualified as a physiotherapist and I as a nurse. When he was not at the hospital he worked repainting walls and fences.

You were born in the same year your father and I met. Your father loved you so much and insisted on taking you everywhere with him. He bought a baby carrier for you and took you around in it. People often made fun of him as a man looking after a baby but he didn't care. Unfortunately in 1989 he and I discovered we had HIV and in 1996 AIDS claimed him. On his final day he told me to take care of you.

family, but it's not enough money to save me from death."

So Christine wasn't taking any medication at all. She said she felt more weary now than she had the previous year. She had been feeling sick for seven years. When her husband suddenly began losing weight and fading away, she knew. The day after her husband died, she went for a test. The result was no surprise. She kept everything to herself for a year. Then she told people, first her sister and then her mother. Whereupon her sister told her that she too was sick.

"I told Aida once she had celebrated her thirteenth birthday. I noticed that the disease was beginning to affect me. It was no longer dormant in my body. It had started moving."

"What did she say?"

"You've asked that already. She said nothing. She was distressed. I believe she already knew that I was sick."

"How could she know that?"

"Aida's a bright girl who listens to what people are saying. And she's not afraid to ask. But most important of all is that she doesn't believe all those people who say that this disease does not even exist."

We had reached the car. The driver was asleep. Flies were buzzing around, there was a smell of crushed banana and wet soil. Christine looked at me.

"You are not surprised? You must know that lots of people, many too many, still think there is no such disease as AIDS. Or else they think it's a disease they can get rid of in various terrible ways."

I nodded, because I did know.

When we drove off, Aida was standing with a huge pan in her hand. Christine waved, as did her mother and other members of the family. Aida didn't wave because she was holding something in her hand. But I knew even then that I would be returning.

How can you sometimes know things you don't know? You just know.

· 16 ·

That evening I thought about what Christine had said. About all those people who still refused to accept that there was such a disease as AIDS. And those who did not deny the existence of the disease, yet maintained that there were strange and wondrous ways of curing it. I remembered a sign I'd seen fifteen years before in Zambia, somewhere between Kabwe and Kapiri Mposhi. "I'll repair your bike while my brother cures you of AIDS."

I thought about what is happening in South Africa right now. The incidence of rapes has been growing for a long time. Until just a few years ago, most of the rape victims were grown women, or at least teenagers. Not any longer. Since 2001, in some parts of the country, there has been an increase in the number of rapes of children, and most repugnant of all: rapes of infants. This has to do with the widespread, lunatic belief that you can be cured of AIDS by having intercourse with a virgin.

How can one fight such crazy ideas? People are desperate. How will it be possible to control the AIDS epidemic if people continue holding such impossible beliefs?

Christine had talked about her work. About her work as a teacher of the next generation.

She said: "Every time I face my class, it's as if my vision becomes blurred. The same as it is with my father's eyes. Sometimes he complains—although he is not the complaining kind—that everything around him seems to be duplicated many times over. He sees ten of me, and just as many of my mother. It's the same with me when I'm standing in front of my pupils. Despite the fact that I don't have a problem with my eyesight. Not yet, anyway, although I know that many people with AIDS go blind before they die. I see my pupils multiply before my eyes. And I see all the children who have not yet become my pupils. All those who will never learn how to read and write. Being able to read and write means being able to survive. How else can you find out how diseases are spread, how else can you learn how to protect yourself and survive? Of course medicines are important, of course I wish my wages were sufficient for my treatment. But it's just as important that all the children I see as blurred images have access to the knowledge that could save them from an all-too-early death. I want them not to have to write memory books for their own children because they die so young."

That is what Christine said. Several times. She wanted me to remember. That's why she kept repeating it.

· 17 ·

Memory books. Writings as death approaches, about death and about life.

This is what this text I am writing is supposed to be about.

I did not go to Uganda so that a girl named Aida would show me the mango plant she tended with such care and concealed under a pile of twigs so that the family's pigs wouldn't gobble it up. I had traveled to Uganda to meet people who were preparing for death by writing little books for their children.

I do not recall the first time I heard about these memory books, but I recognized immediately that they were something I should find out more about. These memory books, small exercise books with glued-in pictures and texts written by people who could barely recite the alphabet, could prove to be the most important documents our time has produced. When all the official reports, minutes, balance sheets, poetry collections, plays, formulas for the control of robots, computer programs, all the archive materials that represent the foundation on which our life and our history is based —when all that has been forgotten, it could be that these slim volumes, these memoirs left behind by human beings who died too soon, prove to be the most significant documents of our epoch.

Five hundred years from now, what will be left from our time and the ages that preceded us? The Greek tragedies, of course, Shakespeare, and a few other things. Most treasures will be lost, and if not completely forgotten, then kept alive only by a tiny minority. But these memory books could well live on and tell future generations about the terrible affliction that affected our age, that killed millions of people and made millions of children orphans.

There were a lot of questions to ask. How does a person tell his or her story when he or she cannot even write? I was exposed to many different types of storytelling. Memories can be smells, drawings; they do not need to be photographs or written texts. What is the essence that tells others who we are? No doubt the diaries of some people will have something to say about me. But what do the words mean? Apart from the fact that I laugh or cry or smell of garlic?

Storytelling involves words. In olden times sto-

You First Talked
When You Were . . .

You first talked when you were 8 months. Everybody in the building kept quiet and listened to you. Your first word was the name of the house girl who used to take care of you. Her name was Emma but you could not pronounce it properly and said "Amma." I remember one time you couldn't find Emma and left the house to look for her. We had to spend half a day looking for you! When you wanted water you could not pronounce the word but said m-uk mu-k instead. Then I would give you water and you would keep quiet.

ries were handed down by word of mouth from generation to generation, and in many parts of the world that is no doubt still true today. But what is to become of the story when so many links in the human chain disappear? What can children say about their parents if they do not remember anything because they were so young when their parents died? Or to put it another way: how can parents explain who they are to children who are so young that they can't comprehend?

This is what memory books are all about.

How does a person tell his story if he cannot write? When he can no longer pass his story by telling it to the next generation? The answer dawned on me. Everybody can tell his or her own story. Words make everything simpler; they are the best method. But it seemed to me that words could be replaced. It must be possible for illiterate people to tell their stories. Smells, imprints, drawings, or perhaps pictures taken by cheap disposable cameras. Why not supply everyone who wanted to leave behind a memory book with one of these single-use cameras? It isn't true, of course, that pictures say more than a thousand words—words usually tell more—but a face, a smile, a body, a person standing in front of a house wall or a clump of banana trees could be just as significant.

This is what memory books are all about: children must be able to tune into their parents who are no longer alive. Recollections of physical contact buried deep down inside, words and voices that are only vague memories, as something in a dream.

·18·

I went to Uganda in order to understand all this, so that I could write about it. In order to be able to tell readers that these memory books, or min-nesskrifter, libros des memorias, errinerungsbücher, livres de mémoires, are important documents of our time.

Important. But at the same time, there should be no need whatsoever for such books to exist. The ultimate objective of the Memory Books program has to be a contribution toward the task of ensuring that one day they will be no longer necessary. Nobody should have to die early from AIDS. The search for vaccines and cures must be continually intensified, and existing antiretroviral (ARV) drugs have to be made accessible to all. Nobody should need to write memory books in the future.

But millions of these memory books still do need to be written. And it goes without saying that everybody should have the right to do so and receive help when they need it. No orphaned child, whether they live in a village north of Kampala or in some village in China or India, should find themselves growing to adulthood knowing nothing about their parents.

Apart from the fact that they died of AIDS.

How many people today in a country like Sweden, my country, know what a terrible disease AIDS is? Have we forgotten already the pictures and descriptions produced ten and fifteen years ago when it was not at all sure whether we would be able to control the epidemic? Those who have the disease know, their relatives know, and the carers who look after them know. But for most other people AIDS is a disease that makes you very thin and fade away, possibly gives you black patches on your face, which leads to the collapse of your immune system, which leads to persistent infections and eventually perhaps fatal pneumonia. All this is correct. But the fact is that AIDS often also involves extreme pain, difficult to alleviate or very difficult to eliminate altogether.

In Sweden, highly qualified and devoted care is available for as long as it is needed. About ten years ago so-called antiretroviral drugs began to appear. It was possible to control HIV because ARVs delay the onset of AIDS. People infected could start to hope that they might be able to live a long life after all. But in a poor country in Africa, where medical care is already primitive? They have to cope with a constant lack of resources—everything from clean sheets to the most advanced medication. And in

You Walked
When You Were . . .

You walked when you were 13 months. You were so tiny. As soon as you could stand up you tried to jump, even before you could walk. And you liked to dance. Your first attempt to play with me involved your pushing me with your head.

such countries, the squeeze on what care and assistance may be made available is all the time increasing. What are the prospects there?

To suffer from AIDS in Sweden and to suffer from AIDS in a country like Uganda are two entirely different things. The gulf between the two peoples is the gulf that lies between the rich and the poor. In all areas. Even when it comes to nursing. Even when it comes to pain.

If you happen to be born in a poor country, the risk of being forced to suffer unimaginable pain is infinitely greater than in a country like Sweden. In a poor country there is a devastating relative lack of resources and the medical capacity to alleviate pain. This is incredibly cruel. If you are doomed to die, the agony you are condemned to endure should not depend on where you happen to be born.

· 19 ·

The day that Christine showed me the memory book she had written for Aida, Aida herself secretly took me to show me her mango plant. The two things were connected, of course: what Christine did and what Aida did. But it was not a prearranged plan. Plans often emerge of their own accord when it comes to death and the sorrow that is in store. Every time the memory book was mentioned, Aida sought consolation in her mango plant. In order to endure the prospect of death she had to make an invocation to life.

·20·

The little memory books follow a basic template. An outline is provided on preprinted pages. There is a simple logic in the headings printed on the various pages. But all the memory books I read in Uganda were original. No two were alike.

People choose their own roads along which to travel. The most important thing is not to follow the manual but to tell about the very special things that only the writer has experienced. They don't need to be told about that. People think like that of their own accord. Everybody knows what is special about themselves, even if most people are modest enough to think they are no more than ordinary. But an ordinary person is always a person with unique and surprising experiences.

·21·

I spent a large part of one of the evenings I was in Uganda thinking about what precisely the memory of a person is. I thought about myself, of course.

What do I want people to remember about me? What would I prefer to have suppressed? Do I have a number of secrets that I will take with me to the grave? How can I shape other people's recollections of me?

It is an impossible task. I can hardly control what anyone else chooses to remember about me. I can only have a vague idea of what sort of an impression I have made. To some extent I can anticipate reactions to what I have written, what I have done in the theater. But what about the memory of me as an individual? The child who was born in St Göran's Hospital in Stockholm at four o'clock in the morning of February 3, 1948?

I can guess that people's memories will vary. Some will remember me as a rather gloomy, possibly even melancholy person who needs to be left in peace and who can flare up if he's disturbed. Others will remember me as the opposite, a decent, cheerful person who will hardly be the last name to spring to mind when drawing up a guest list for a party.

I don't know what people will remember. Nor for how long. Memories are always finite. Memories of me will last for a number of years, but the day will come when they no longer survive. It is given to very few to live on beyond the memories of their grandchildren. After a hundred years most of us are one of the anonymous gray shadows in the blackness that surrounds us all.

But I also turn the question around: what do I remember about others?

That evening in Kampala I lay in the darkness and thought about my own parents. That was only natural. Obviously, they were important to me when I was growing up. But in quite different ways. My father was the one I lived with. Without his ability to notice me, listen, be positive, I don't know how I would have turned out. He more than made up for the fact that my mother was present only through her absence. She didn't exist except as a figure in photographs that were hidden away and kept from me. My mother was a strange shadow when I was little. I can't remember how old I was when it finally dawned on me that there was something peculiar about my mother. But I remember asking my paternal grandmother, who lived with us, why I didn't have a mother. I don't recall her answer, but it was evasive, I did notice that. That is something children learn at an early age—how to interpret the way adults answer questions. They soon learn how to tune their antennae to distinguish between the truth and a lie, what is a clear answer, and what is evasive.

Then, when I was six, I started searching in secret for traces of this mother of mine who had disappeared. I found several photographs. Including one of me sitting on her knee. They were taken in a photographer's studio on my first birthday. I can still remember my heart pounding when I saw my mother's face for the first time. She had disappeared at such an early stage that I had no memory of her. Now I could see what she looked like. I was surprised that she was so unlike my father. Didn't people who had children have to look like each other? Then it struck me that in the photograph she was looking at me as if I were a child she didn't know. A changeling or something the fairies had brought.

I don't know that I thought that at the time, of course, or that it was so well formulated. But I doubtless realized that there was something funny about the photograph. She was holding me as if I were a burden she would like to put down as swiftly as possible.

In Kampala that night I thought about her and my father, both of them now long since dead. I had difficulty in conjuring up their faces in the darkness. That was a shocking moment. I had forgotten what my parents looked like. It had been a long time since I had seen them, of course: my father died in April 1972 and my mother a couple of years later. There was a no-man's-land of thirty years between the faces I had seen and those I could no longer remember.

On the other hand I could quite distinctly recall

When You Were Little
You Loved to . . .

You loved to go for unannounced visits, especially to see your grandmother. You loved to go out with me and to play outside. I remember when we went to Children's Lunar Park. The first ride you went on was a little car and then you went on a swing. You wanted me to spend all our money on the swings. I also remember that you had a Kamba cassette and that you danced to it in your own style. Watching you dance just made me love you all the more. You were always asking me when I would buy you a car. When I told you my parents had a car you wanted to know whether we could borrow it so that I could give you a ride.

the smell of my father's hair and his suits. My mother's face was blurred, but I could remember the sound of her voice, the way she spoke, the unmistakable traces of the Örebro dialect that she had spoken as a child.

In my mind I wrote a few memory books about my parents. And of course it was possible to do that. The memories of a smell and a voice meant that the faces slowly came out of the darkness. Now I could see my parents again. The memories behind those smells and sounds opened up many other avenues of memory. I recalled events, conversations, images, both in close-up and long shots.

It is true that neither words nor photographic images are necessary for memories. That is precisely why the examples of memory books that I saw in Uganda were so remarkable. I thumbed through the little exercise books. They contained pressed flowers, insects, one including a butterfly whose wings gleamed in an unusual shade of blue. Somebody had Scotch-taped in grains of sand. There were also drawings: matchstick men, landscapes, animals, as if the pages were ancient cave paintings.

I saw stories without words, without pictures. There was joy and clarity in these stories. But, inevitably, mainly despair and worry: what will happen to my children when I have gone? All those I spoke to, all the people who had overcome their uncertainties and produced memory books for their children were pleased they had done so. I talked to men and women, all of whom had made nine or ten stories, one for each of their children, told in different ways because the children were of different ages.

Stories are bridges. Nobody regrets the building of a bridge.

Needless to say, that was the most moving and at the same time the most poignant aspect of these slim little memory books. They were farewells, inexorable farewell letters. All the stories ended up in an infinite emptiness; they were about lives that would end far too soon.

Christine said as much very clearly in reply to one of my questions: "When does death come too soon?"

She thought for a long time before answering.

"When does a person die too soon? There are lots of different answers to that. One answer that is always true is: when a parent, usually a mother, is forced to leave her children when they are too small to take care of themselves. And when she cannot be sure that someone else can be counted upon to take care of her children when she has gone."

Suddenly she realized that some of her children were listening. She fell silent immediately.

"Do you think they can hear what we're talking about?"

"I don't know."

Then she burst out laughing.

"It doesn't matter. Why should I try to fool myself or my children or my friends? Everybody knows my time is limited."

Later, our last day together, she returned to the question:

"Death always makes a mess of things, no matter when it comes."

·23·

I've experienced this before.

People who are shortly going to die want to know that they are still alive. Often with a desperate and at times ferocious intensity.

Once I had a friend who had bone cancer. To the very end he suppressed the fact that he was in great pain and had only months to live. He wouldn't even reach forty. We had known each other for a long time. The sad thing was, he had always imagined that when he retired, he would sail around the world. One day when I went to see him he insisted on examining his face in a mirror and then asked me if I thought his face had grown more mature-looking in recent years. I agreed with him, naturally. Now, many years after he died, I can't remember talking about anything else on that occasion, just that his face had grown more mature and signaled a man on the way to his prime.

That's how it was too with the people with AIDS that I met in the villages north of Kampala. They showed me things all the time. Photographs, a newly painted room, a knitted sweater. Everything was significant because they thought it confirmed their existence, was a sign that they were still alive. They were somehow protected by these objects. Despite the fact that many of them were already so acutely ill that they would very soon die, the objects gave them the illusion of being a safe distance away from cold death.

· 24 ·

During my visit to Uganda I spoke with a lot of sick people, but I spoke most often with Christine, Gladys, and Moses. And there was also Aida, the girl who wasn't ill, the girl who wasn't going to die but instead would have to take on huge responsibilities.

The girl who was nurturing a mango plant.

I have already written about Christine. A few miles from her house lived Moses. I had made a few notes on the overnight flight from London, but when I looked at them later, the questions I had written seemed idiotic. The most idiotic of all was: "When did you start being afraid?"

It was the most obvious question, of course. Fear, open or concealed, affects everybody suffering from a fatal disease. You keep waiting for test results that can turn out to be a death sentence.

A young man who tested positive for HIV in Gothenburg at the end of the 1980s told me how the doctor who had to inform him of the positive result burst into tears. He was nineteen when he discovered that he was infected. Instead of trying to cope with his own fear, he found himself having to console the weeping doctor.

When did you start being afraid?

When had I been afraid?

During the night I spent on the flight from London to Entebbe, I thought a lot about the occasions in my life when I had been paralyzed with fear. I could recall three situations in particular, one of them when I was waiting for news from a doctor.

I was in Mozambique, it was autumn, the days were hot. I was working on the production of a play but started to feel unwell. I suspected it was influenza, possibly malaria, or it could simply be exhaustion. As usual, I had been working far too many hours. The tiredness wouldn't go away. I dragged myself as far as my Renault 4 in the mornings and sat there, having long, silent conversations with myself before making up my mind to try to work one more day.

But then one morning, when I reached the theater and parked the car, I stayed behind the wheel. It was obvious that there was something badly wrong with me. I was seriously ill; something nasty

Your Favorite Book, Game, Cartoon Character, and TV Show Were . . .

Your favorite games were football and hide and seek. As for TV, you liked the shows Maria de Los Angeles, Vituko, Vioja Mahakawan, Bold and Beautiful, Tom and Jerry cartoons, and wrestling. And on the radio you listened to Kayu Ka Miungi FM. You often walked around singing to KKM.

You often insisted I buy video tapes of action movies featuring stars like Chuck Norris, but you always ran away when a fight broke out in the film. I remember one time you jumped into the compound and told me a boy was threatening to beat you. You didn't like to fight and you took no chances with other boys. You were small and humble. The neighborhood loved you.

had found its way into my body and was threatening my life. I drove home again, but stopped on the way to buy some food. As I went up the steps I bumped into Christer, a Swedish dentist and aid worker.

"You're completely yellow," he said.

I went to my doctor, who sent me to a clinic for tests, and I returned with liver readings that were nothing short of catastrophic. I was sent at once to South Africa. I remember nothing of the journey. But it was an aggressive form of jaundice. (I suspect it was caused by a dirty salad at a restaurant in Pemba in northern Mozambique.)

But it wasn't only jaundice. One morning a doctor came to see me. He was obese and was wearing a yarmulke. I remember my messengers over the years very clearly, all the people who have passed on to me vital information.

I did not know his name, but I remember there was sweat on his forehead as he told me, without beating around the bush, that they had found a patch on one of my lungs. It could be ominous. It would take several days for all the test results to come back. Then he went away. I don't think he had looked me in the eye once during the brief time he was in my room.

I remember the feeling of paralysis that gripped me. Panic was a sharp hook stabbing into my consciousness and immediately sending signals to all parts of my body. Fear makes itself felt in the stomach as well as in the brain. It was like a frantic telegram being rattled out by a machine inside me.

Lung cancer. I hadn't avoided it.

I smoked my first cigarette at Spencer's Café in Borås, in Allégatan. It must have been one of the last days in August 1963. I had just started secondary school. One of my classmates, a girl called Hedelin I think it was, offered me a cigarette. A Prince. I had never smoked before, apart from a couple of furtive puffs on stumps of cigars in Sveg. But now I felt obliged to accept the cigarette. From then on I was a smoker. Although I had long since stopped smoking by the time that doctor came into my room, all those packs of cigarettes had caught up with me. Followed me all the way down to southern Africa. I had stopped smoking too late. Lung cancer was going to kill me. I could envisage my lungs covered in lumps of tar. In desperation, trying as much as possible to keep my panic under control, I tried to convince myself that I might be able to live for a few more years. Not more than a few, probably, but long enough to have a chance to complete some of the things I had planned. Not ten books, but maybe two. And a play, if I really worked hard.

Then followed a few days of extreme panic. I lay in my sickroom, sometimes listening to the sound of gunfire in the unsettled Johannesburg night; the fear came and went in waves. I don't recall ever starting to cry, though. I stopped short of that. It would be a defeat already if I went to pieces. In that case the illness would be let loose and finish me off immediately. I tried to imagine the number of days in which I would be able to lead a normal life in spite of everything. I tried to convince myself that the cancer had been discovered very early and hence I would have a considerable way to go before my last journey.

I lay awake at night, hoping the whole thing might be a mistake. A technical fault in the X-ray machine, a piece of dust on the plate.

One morning the obese doctor with the yarmulke came back. I gripped the bed frame tightly and prepared to listen to my death sentence. But he informed me that it was an accumulation of fluid in one of my lungs. Nothing dangerous, not cancer, nothing to worry about. Then he was gone.

I wonder what he knew about people's fear. Perhaps it was beneath his dignity to worry about such lowly human emotional reactions? I thought afterwards, and I still feel that I hate that man for his inability to recognize my fear. But what about me? Do I see the fear of others when it should be obvious?

Both my other two moments of well-founded terror are associated with incidents in Africa. Late one night in Lusaka I was attacked as I parked my car outside the house where I lived. I was dragged out of the car by a man with bloodshot, drug-crazed eyes. He held a pistol to my head. I still don't know how long it was there. I have tried to reconstruct how long it would have taken the bandits to pull me from the car. Thirty seconds? More? Less? I don't know. But I was quite certain that I was about to die. Most often in Zambia in the 1980s the car hijackers did shoot. They had nothing to lose. If anyone used a gun in the course of a robbery, it was a hanging offense. And hanged they were. Absurdly enough, the hangman in Zambia was called White, as I recall it. Anyway, it was usual practice for the hijackers to shoot. I remember the cold terror, as if somebody were slowly filling my veins with liquid ice. I was sure that I was about to die, and that I didn't want to die in this stupid, barbaric way. Then the revolver was taken away, I was kicked to the ground, and as the car drove off with a racing start it came to me that I was still alive.

The third moment was the worst. It might seem exotic, almost comical, but it was the most dangerous thing to have happened to me in my life. (Nobody knows, of course, how close one might have been to a plane crash or a road accident.)

It was on one of the little tributaries of the River Kabompo in Zambia, still in the 1980s. There were several of us on a fishing trip. We cruised up the river, switched off the engine, and started fishing as we drifted. We knew that there was a colony of hippos just past a point where the river split into two branches, some way downstream in the direction we were drifting toward. In good time before we reached there, we would start the engine again and turn off along the other branch. Hippos are extremely dangerous if they think their calves are under threat. And these hippos had young. Some distance before we reached the colony, one of us pulled at the cord to start the outboard motor. Nothing happened. At first there was no panic. The man in the stern kept pulling, adjusted the choke, tried again. No ignition. By now we could see the heads of the hippos. We didn't need to say anything, but we all knew that if the engine didn't start, we wouldn't stand a chance. The hippos would attack the boat, overturn it, and then hack us to pieces with their enormous jaws. There would be no point in diving into the river and swimming for it. Not one of us would reach the bank—the river was teeming with crocodiles.

At the last possible moment the engine gave a cough and started. There must have been an angel in the carburetor.

What I remember now, so many years later, is the relief I felt as the boat moved away. We never referred to the incident afterwards. If I remember correctly, we continued fishing.

· 25 ·

But there was also the time I took an HIV test. It was in the mid-1980s, when everybody still felt insecure. Despite all the assurances about how the virus was passed on, was there a possibility that it could infect people in some other way? Nobody could be certain, and opinions were divided on whether kisses could be infectious or not. In other words, there was a gray area around the assertion that HIV was a weak virus, could survive only for about twenty minutes at room temperature, and therefore it was not so easy to become infected and one could avoid it by simple precautionary measures.

I took a test at the hospital in Ystad. The doctor asked me why I was doing this and I said I had no reason to believe that I had been infected, but that I was doing it "for safety's sake." He had no objection. I suspected that he had probably undergone tests himself, just "for safety's sake."

Afterward, when I had had my blood sample taken and registered, when I was on my way home in the car, I suddenly felt scared. I was so shaken that I had to pull over. It was a wet day in the autumn. I got out of the car and felt quite certain that the result of the test would be positive. Nobody, least of all me, would ever be able to explain how it had happened. Perhaps I would be the first one to demonstrate that there really was a very large gray area blurring the convictions of medical science regarding how the disease was passed on.

The three days that followed were pure nightmare. Common sense told me that I had nothing to worry about. But I jumped every time the telephone rang. I woke up each night and stared into the darkness.

The nurse duly phoned on the third day. A shiver ran down my spine when she said who she was. But, predictably, I was not summoned back to the hospital. She simply told me, with no appearance of feeling, that the test result was negative. I thanked her for informing me, perfectly calmly, with no trace of stress, and replaced the receiver.

Then I went out into the rain and fell to my knees in the mud. I stayed like that for a long time before going back indoors. My relief had been manically exaggerated. Not joy, just relief. I can still remember the mud clinging to my trouser legs.

I had been afraid for no reason. What must it be like for those who take the test and know that there really is a risk that he or she has been infected?

· 26 ·

Moses was the only man with whom I had real conversations during my stay in Uganda. Beatrice, who worked with people with HIV, told me that men seldom write memory books. Nor were they so willing to talk about their fate, whereas women were always prepared to talk openly about their

You Didn't Like to Eat . . .

You didn't like meat and I always worried that that contributed to your poor health. Generally, you used to enjoy playing more than eating. But when I pointed out to you that this was a problem you always listened to me and tried to understand. One item of food you loved was cake. Once, on your birthday, you whispered to me that I should not share your cake with the friends and cousins who were at your party.

lives. But there were exceptions, and Moses was only one of many, even though for various reasons he was the only one I ended up talking to.

The last time I spoke to him somebody took a couple of photographs with a Polaroid camera that I had with me. Moses and I are sitting on a couple of wooden stools in the shade of a tree. He kept one of the pictures, I kept the other. Whenever I look at it I wonder how he is, if he's still alive, if he's in pain. And I think that the picture shows him exactly as I remember him. A face radiating great dignity. A man who has accepted that life can suddenly change course, and nothing will ever be the same again.

Moses lived not far from Christine. He had a large family; several of his children had families of their own and some lived in the same house as he did. He sat in the shade, pointing out all his grandchildren and telling me their names and ages; he characterized their "lust for life" in various ways. One of them, a girl, delighted in kicking a homemade football around their yard. A boy, aged about ten, could climb any tree that stood in his path. He could climb as high as you like, as quick as a flash. That was the way he liked to characterize his grandchildren, and he would keep laughing out loud. But much of the time he was melancholy.

He had written about fifteen memory books, one for each of his children and some for the older grandchildren. He didn't tell me how he had caught the virus, but his two wives were dead; no doubt he had infected them, and they had both died before him. I thought several times that I should ask him. But I never managed to overcome my hesitation. And now it's too late.

I asked him about the memory books.

"Somebody told me about them. Beatrice. At first I thought they weren't for me, but I couldn't get them out of my mind. One day I went to that center where people who have the disease can go for help and advice. I spoke to another man who was also ill. He showed me a memory book he had written for one of his daughters. That made me think I should do the same. Even if I'm not very good at writing. I thought I could tell the tale, and one of my grandchildren could write it down. All of them can read and write. So that's what I did."

We leafed through one of the memory books he'd written. All the text was in rounded, childish letters. Everything except his signature and an admonition to "always live honorably and work hard."

He noticed that I could see the text had been written by various hands.

"I thought that even handwriting is a memory of a person. My handwriting is poor, the letters jump all over the place, but it's my handwriting. When I'm gone, my grandchildren can remember that this is how their grandfather used to write."

Then he started talking about how the fatal disease that had taken possession of his body had crept up on him.

"It came in the night. Illness never strikes when the sun is shining. Diseases, especially those that are serious and kill or blind or deform people, always creep up on you during the night."

I asked him what he meant by that.

"The mosquitoes start whining at night. They only suck your blood from sundown until the sun starts rising again. Mosquitoes carry death, malaria. Snakes and predators also roam in the hours of darkness, even if we haven't had any lions or leopards in these parts for the last ten or even fifteen years. We are convinced that disease strikes you during the night."

"A bite in the neck from a leopard can hardly be called a disease!"

"Everything that kills, be it visible or invisible, is a disease as far as I'm concerned. I know that you Europeans talk about something you call 'death from natural causes.' For us Africans that is a very peculiar way of looking at what happens in the dark."

But then he suddenly seemed to have lost interest in discussing his view that the night is the realm of death and illness. Instead he started talking about when he first realized that there was a new disease that was dangerous and invisible.

He had just started talking when the heavens opened. We took cover and sat in a part of the large house that he had to himself. One of his daughters, Laurentina, was very fat but moved gracefully and quickly despite her huge body. When we came in, she disappeared behind a curtain made from old cut-up skirts. It was dim inside the room. Moses sat down in a sagging armchair from which he could keep an eye on what was happening outside while he spoke.

He said: "I was still very young. It was 1974, the year before Amin came to power and ruined our country. My father often used to go to Kampala to buy cheap clothes with factory faults that he fixed and then bicycled through the villages and sold them. One day he came home and told us about one of the young men he used to do business with in the city: he was now ill. My father said he had grown very thin in a very short space of time. He had lost his appetite, the glands under his arms had swollen up and were very tender, and now he was getting sores all over his body. He had been to the doctor, who had been unable to tell him what he was suffering from, nor could he give him any effective medicine. My father was quite sure about what he was saying. He had a keen eye, a good memory, and he often was quite certain about things before anybody else realized that something had happened. That was exactly what he said: 'Something has happened.' His business contact, Lukas was his name, was suffering from a disease that my father was convinced was something quite new. 'It has crept up in the night,' my father said. Lukas died, and his two wives also fell ill and had the same mysterious sores, and one after the other they too died. Every time my father came back from Kampala, he told us about other people who had died from this same disease. Soon, so many had fallen victim to the disease that everybody was talking about why people all of a sudden became very tired and very thin and then died. But nobody knew what it was. I think that was the situation until the 1980s—in any case Amin was no longer around when the disease was finally given a name and it was understood how the infection could be spread. I was no longer so young by then. My father lived to be very old, and of course he was not surprised to find that he had eventually been proved right. What his friend Lukas had died of was a new disease that had crept up on us during the night. He had noticed it before anybody else."

Moses fell silent. Then he shouted something to his daughter. She came in with a bottle of water and two glasses. Moses poured, and assured me that the water had been boiled.

"It is a terrible plague," he said after a while. "In the night, in the darkness, when men and women come together, the disease wanders from person to person. There have been other diseases in the past that have infected people in the same way. But nothing as dangerous as this, nothing as painful. I have seen how people suffer before they die. I have

I Always Laughed When You . . .

I used to laugh when you asked, as you often did, when your birthday was coming up. This was especially funny—I knew the only reason you wanted it to be your birthday was because there would be cake at the party. You were always asking me "Did you get my birthday cake yet?"

Another occasion I recall laughing was when you came home from school and proudly announced that you were 35th in your class and had beaten your friend who was only number one. I tried to explain to you that being first was better than being thirty-fifth but you would have none of it—for you, the more the better.

listened to people in houses a long way away from here, screaming in agony before everything goes quiet, and they fade away into the other darkness, the one that never quite dissipates when the sun rises again. The land of death is a land without sun, that is the nature of it and we are all frightened of being forced to go there before we have lived for so long that we don't really care any more. Now I have the disease myself, and every day I look for signs to show that I am on the way to being overcome by this thing inside me, and every time I think about that day my father came home and was worried as he told us about his friend Lukas."

Moses stared at his hands.

"I didn't want to write these memory books. Not for a very long time. It was as if the moment I picked up my pen or started telling my story for my grandchildren to write it down, I was giving up all hope of not having to die as a result of this disease. Obviously, I don't have any hope. Everybody who catches this disease dies of it. But deep down there is another kind of hope, something you have no control over. It's as if there is an unknown being inside my body that is hoping on my behalf. I don't know how to explain it any better than that. But once I'd started to write those books, it was as if I'd accepted the fact that I was going to die. I dreamed about my father the night before I started preparing to write the memory books. He was coming back from the city on foot, just as I remembered it as a child. He always walked quickly, carrying a bale of clothes on his head. Now he was old and didn't have anything on his head. The worst thing was that he didn't stop. He didn't turn off the road and come back here. He just kept on walking until I could no longer see him. When I woke up the next morning and remembered the dream, it seemed as if he had instructed me to accept my fate. That was the day I started preparing the books."

Moses had finished his tale abruptly, as if he'd told me too big a secret. Then he said with a smile that he was tired, and needed to rest.

We said our good-byes, and I left. I didn't know if I would ever meet him again.

· 27 ·

Lots of people have jokes to tell about the AIDS crisis on the African continent. Some even try to use various anecdotes in order to prove that the basic problem is the inability of Africans to absorb information. Many ignore the fact that the real problem is illiteracy. Instead, these unpleasant jokesmiths conjure up an image of stupidity, a peculiar lack of intelligence when faced with facts and arguments. The stories and the conclusions are downright racist. The implication is that it is the natives' own fault that so many Africans are HIV-positive. They ought to know better than indulge in extramarital affairs or lead polygamous lives. If they are infected, there is not much that can be done about it. Let them die.

This is not said in so many words, of course. But I have heard the joke, told by a Scandinavian aid worker, about the European nurse who traveled to a remote African village to address them on the subject of AIDS. She talked about condoms. To demonstrate how they should be used she stuck up two fingers and slid the condom over them. Whereupon all the men present, according to the Scandinavian teller of the tale, went home and applied a condom to their fingers before having sex with their wives.

It is easy to make fun, racist fun, of African people. But misunderstandings about safe sex are not a result of stupidity. They are a relic of the tradition and heritage that Europeans have forced upon Africa. They have to do with the only golden rule that mattered during the four centuries of colonialism. Europe said: don't think, do!

Unsurprisingly, this attitude lingers on. It is neither stupidity nor cowardice. It is a continuation of European pressure. Moreover, teaching people how to protect themselves is a very sensitive matter. In many African cultures you simply do not talk to strangers about your intimate sex life. It is completely inappropriate for a clumsy European to march up and gather villagers together, then make threatening gestures with his or her fingers and slide a condom over them. Being illiterate is not the same thing as being devoid of dignity.

I have met vast numbers of poor, ignorant Africans whose dignity far exceeds anything I have come across in the West. This is not a tendentious or far-fetched claim. Human dignity does not go arm-in-arm with material well-being or a high degree of knowledge. Human dignity is an automatic reaction in poor people who have understood why they are weighed down by poverty.

Informing people about how the infection is passed on is crucial, obviously, but the teaching has to be adapted to those who are to be taught. Those whose mission it is to impart this information must first learn to listen, and not seek to impose the solutions and rules of conduct that various Western experts and bureaucrats have decided are correct.

Thousands of people are dying of AIDS today because of wrong, often downright arrogant methods of trying to make them realize how HIV is transmitted. There is no doubt that one essential tool in the effort to reduce the rate of infection, whether in young or rather older people, would be taking steps to ensure that everybody has access to an alphabet book. For instance.

The statistics paint a complex picture, but they tell the same story. It is a lack of basic education that makes people more vulnerable to HIV infection.

There was one question that I asked everybody I talked to in Uganda. A question I had also asked people earlier in Mozambique, people suffering from full-blown AIDS, or people who had just been infected and told that they were carrying HIV.

I asked them where they thought the virus had come from.

Replies varied. Astonishingly, many thought that it could very well be a disease the West had introduced secretly into Africa, and was making sure that it spread everywhere in order to reduce the number of poor people there. In other words, the disease was a subtle way of committing mass murder. The invisible gas chambers of a new age, a microscopic virus that could send people to their graves in a "natural" way. People who believed this to be the origin of the HIV epidemic often replied very emphatically. They were absolutely convinced that the death they were facing had been deliberately planned. The whole of the West was made up of witches or medicine men bent on genocide.

There were some who introduced a religious dimension into their fate. Abandoned gods were spreading death and destruction all over an Africa that already seemed to be ripe for extinction.

I Always Remember the Time . . .

I remember when I told you I didn't have money to buy you the books you needed for school and you consoled me and told me we could get by without them, that you could borrow them from the school.

I also remember when I told you about my having HIV. You stood firm and told me that maybe God would heal me. I have never forgotten the hope I saw in your eyes then. It was rekindled every morning when we said goodbye before you left for school. You always hugged and kissed me and said "Misssss Nighhhht" to me. That was exactly what you said.

I recall that once you burnt your fingers quite severely and you asked me whether I couldn't ask Jesus to give you new hands. You were perfectly serious but I laughed and I told you that was not possible. You insisted on knowing why.

And I remember on the night of the millennium you wanted to see the New Year arrive. You stayed out until 1:30 in the morning and then returned miserable, telling me that you hadn't seen anything at all. I took a lot of time trying to explain to you that the New Year was only a matter of time passing from 12:00 to 12:01. Even then I don't think you understood.

Famine, civil war, expanding deserts, malaria parasites, and diarrhea. And now AIDS. There was a self-disgust about these people that doubled their suffering. They were often the ones who lived for the shortest time. Their immune system was unable to cope with the double pressure of the ravages caused by the virus and their mental collapse.

These people gave the impression of using the virus as a means of committing suicide.

Most others knew nothing more than what the doctors had told them. A virus—whatever that is. Something that resulted from making love, from blood transfusions, or from using dirty syringe needles.

Everybody seemed to agree that the suffering was hitting the African continent especially hard.

Christine said: "It's as if there's no end to it. I read about our continent. It is as if we Africans are concerned only with dying, not with living. But it's not like that, of course. Even if all these diseases hit us especially hard."

Of course there were many people who also maintained that the West was conspiring in some remarkable way with various gods. The overworld and the underworld had combined to destroy the African people with the help of this virus.

Christine again: "I've heard that some people think the disease originated in animals, especially the apes, and that we got the disease inside us when we ate meat from apes. But couldn't it just as well be that we have always carried the disease inside us? Maybe it has always been inside us but it is only now that it has been given a name."

What did Moses think? He shrugged.

"Is it important? I can't tell you the answer—nobody can. Why should I spend my time worrying about that? My time is already limited. Death is wherever there is life. Death sometimes wears visible clothing, sometimes he makes himself invisible."

I spoke to everybody, including Gladys and Beatrice. The answers varied, but were always evasive.

· 29 ·

In the end I spoke to Aida as well. We were in among the banana trees, but not to look at her mango plant: we were trying to find one of the black piglets that had decided to run away. Aida found it and pounced on it before it had a chance to escape her grasp. We carried it back to the pen. Then Aida went to wash her hands.

It was she who asked the question: "Where does it come from, this disease that Mom has?"

"I don't know. Different people think different things. But it's a virus, a so-called microorganism."

"Why is it only people here who get it?"

"It isn't only here. People get infected just the same in the country I come from."

Aida thought about that.

"Where did it start? In your country or here in ours?"

"Probably here, but nobody knows for certain."

Aida seemed depressed. We walked back to the houses and the courtyard, where a cockerel with an injured leg was limping around.

"I think the disease comes from somebody who wants to harm us," Aida suddenly said.

"Who would that be?"

"I don't know."

"Diseases don't come from 'somebody.' Diseases are there all the time. They develop and change. Eventually people start to die of them. It has always been like that."

Aida said nothing more. As we walked towards the raffia mat where Christine sat cleaning a wound on Aida's youngest sister's foot, she aimed a kick at the cockerel who fluttered away, cackling angrily.

Aida could get at the cockerel, but not at the "somebody" she thought had inflicted the disease on her mother.

But I can't be certain what Aida believed or didn't believe.

· 30 ·

There are many fallacies about AIDS. Not least
with regard to what happens in the critical stages
that lead to death—what is known as "full-blown"
AIDS. One of the fallacies is that the really horrific aspect of the disease is the way it strikes in a hap-
hazard fashion, and often affects very young people. What creates angst in a person is the psycho-
logical torment of knowing that you are going to
die early from a disease that you could have avoided. The physical symptoms as the disease takes
hold are that you lose a lot of weight, grow very
tired, might have a lot of sores, and then die of
something like pneumonia when your immune system can no longer cope. There is rarely any men-
tion of the fact that AIDS can lead to a mental
deterioration that causes suffering worse than practically anything else.

The people I spoke to in Uganda seemed to be
aware of this, however. They didn't hide behind fallacies even if the illusion might have been a temporary consolation. It seemed to me that Moses,
Christine, Gladys, and all the rest approached what
was in store for them with their eyes wide-open. It
was a duel they had already lost. Once again it was
that dignity that I couldn't help but notice everywhere, and that I think of now above all else as I

write these words. The dignity that was so important to all those who had been infected with the disease.

On one occasion we met, I told Christine a story. It was about something I experienced in the early 1990s in northern Mozambique. A few days later when I went back to her house, she asked me to tell her the story again. This time Aida was there too.

It was a story about dignity.

During the long and difficult civil war that ravaged Mozambique—from the early 1980s until 1992—I made a journey to the Cabo Delgado province in the north. One day in November 1990, I was in a place just south of the border with Tanzania. The area had been badly affected by the war. Many people had been killed or crippled, and starvation was widespread since most of the crops had been burnt. It was like entering an inferno where misery rose like smoke all along the dusty roads.

One day I took a path that led to a tiny village. A young man came walking toward me. It seemed as if he were walking out of the sun. His clothes were in tatters. He could have been nineteen, maybe twenty. When he came closer, I noticed his feet. I saw something I will never forget as long as I live. I can see it before my very eyes as I am telling this tale now. Rarely does a day pass when I don't think about this boy who was coming towards me as if from out of the sun. What did I see? His feet.

I Hope You Never
Forget the Time . . .

I hope you never forget when you were involved in
the launch of Network of People Living with AIDS.
You presented flowers to the American Ambassador
Bushnell. I also presented a red ribbon to the
Ambassador to mark the good work of the HIV/AIDS
campaigns.

He had painted shoes onto his feet. He had mixed paint from the soil and preserved his dignity for as long as possible. He had no boots, no shoes, nothing, not even a pair of sandals made from the remains of a car tire. As he had no shoes, he had to make some himself, so he painted a pair of shoes onto his feet, and in doing so he boosted his awareness that, despite all his misery and destitution, he was a human being with dignity.

I thought at the time and I still think now that of all the strangers I have met in my life, this meeting may have been the most important of all. For what he told me with his feet was that human dignity can be preserved and maintained when all else seems lost. I learned that we should all be aware that there could come a day when we too will have to paint shoes onto our feet. And when that day comes, it is important that we know that we possess that ability. I don't know what his name was. He couldn't speak Portuguese and I didn't understand his language. I have often wondered what became of him. He is most probably dead, though I have no way of knowing for sure. But the image of his feet will always be with me.

It was like telling a fairy tale, I thought. But Christine knew it was true. She turned to Aida.

"Do you understand what he is talking about?" she asked.

Aida nodded. But she didn't say anything. And

Christine didn't push her to provide an answer, like the sensible mother she was.

· 31 ·

I've seen it once. A person's face just after being told that she has tested positive. But I didn't see it just in her face. The pain and the shock was all over her body. Her feet were screaming, her arms were flailing desperately so as not to go berserk, despite the fact that they were hanging down by her sides.

It was a woman, and she can't have been more than twenty. It was in Maputo, in a private clinic of the simpler kind. I was there to check my blood pressure. I waited outside the closed door to the doctor's consulting room. It opened and the woman emerged. I knew immediately even though I didn't know: this young African woman had just been told that she was HIV-positive. She was just setting out on life, but had found that her time had been brutally cut short. Her life was coming to an end almost before it had started.

She walked away down the corridor. When they measured my blood pressure it was extremely high. The doctor frowned. But I told him it was only temporary. Something had happened shortly before I entered his room that had forced my blood pressure up. Now it was on its way down again.

I keep some people very close at hand, easily accessible in my memory. Aida is one, that nameless woman is another. I very often wonder what became of her, whether she is still alive.

· 32 ·

There was once a famous library in Alexandria. It contained the sum of human wisdom, or as much of it as was recorded, on its shelves. Then it burned down. Now, a few months before I go to Uganda, I pay a visit to the newly opened library in Alexandria. Architecturally, it is a remarkable creation. More of a cultural center than a straightforward library. At the time of my visit an Austrian symphony orchestra is rehearsing in one of the halls.

While I am in Uganda it occurs to me that if all the memory books that are now being written could be gathered together, they might fill the library in Alexandria. There are so many memories to be written down, so many million little books to be left behind after the people who will shortly die from AIDS. The vast majority of these millions of people will die too young. Most of their lives will be cut unjustly short. Many of their children, who are going to receive these books and are the reason why they are being written, will have been made homeless and will end up wandering aimlessly from continent to continent.

Then I have a vision: empty, abandoned libraries, and the great collections of books find themselves with no readers.

It is not a totally outrageous thought. Many a plot could be composed that would be just the thing for a science-fiction movie. There is already research predicting that certain countries or regions in Africa south of the Sahara will be ruined if AIDS continues to spread at the rate it is today. What they say should be taken seriously. The social fabric will be altered. A large percentage of the workforce will be wiped out, making society increasingly dependent on child labor. To make things yet worse, the whole existing intellectual heritage will be in danger of dying out because young people who are infected will not be able to find the motivation for their studies.

Wilderness, child labor, silence. Many people refuse to believe that this could happen. Or at least think it is a threat that won't concern us for a very long time to come. But it takes only about nine hours to fly from the heart of Europe to the heart of Africa. In other words, after a good night's sleep or a somewhat extended working day, and you are in the center of what is threatening to become a wasteland, a return to the most primitive circumstances for work and property.

Some are already commenting on this in their memory books. There are people who are about to die but who do nevertheless try to see into the future. They can comprehend the consequences of their own death, magnified and on a global scale. If there is one thing that is certain when it comes to AIDS in Africa, it is that you will not die alone. Also it is true that your death will have very far-reaching consequences.

I read about this in several of the memory books. The fear of impoverishment, the fear that children will be left to their own devices, the fear that all knowledge will be forgotten and rot away like the dead body of a human being.

AIDS has to do with many kinds of death. Hence also with many kinds of life. Obviously, life can be assessed and interpreted in the number of books that are written and the books that are read.

In 1343, Petrarch found a voluminous manu-script in Verona containing Cicero's letters to his son Atticus: for many years the boy was an idle and unenthusiastic student in Athens. Those letters had been lost since Cicero's time, since the beginning of our chronology. After thirteen hundred years they suddenly reappeared.

Is this what will happen to all the memory books that are being written today? It seems hard-ly credible that in our day and age it would be pos-sible to bury the written word in archives, even as we bury nuclear waste in caverns deep inside mountains. But you never know.

There was once a great library in Alexandria. It contained all of human knowledge until it burned down. Now it has been rebuilt.

Perhaps that library should be a center for all the memory books that are being written today. Perhaps at least copies should be kept there, for the future.

· 33 ·

In the diary I kept during my visit to Uganda there is a stray sentence scribbled down on the inside of the back cover.

"The pain can be seen in their smiles."

Strangely enough, I have to admit that I can't remember when I wrote that. Who had I met? Whose smiles was I referring to? It seems to me odd that I can't remember. I would hardly have made a note like that without good reason.

I scour my memory, but I cannot find the occasion or the cause.

How can I remember a smile without remembering the face?

It wasn't until my last visit to Gladys that I realized that there was a link between her and Christine that I had not known about. Gladys told me when I first visited her that when she heard she had tested HIV-positive, she sat down and stayed sitting down for several years, doing nothing, only waiting to die. On that occasion, I overlooked the obvious question: what shook you out of that apathy?

It was Christine who persuaded her to abandon her apathetic wait for death.

Gladys and Christine knew each other only slightly, but Christine had heard that Gladys was sitting in her dark room as if paralyzed. She never went out, hardly spoke to her children. She just sat there motionless, waiting for the cold breeze on the back of her neck.

One day Christine went to see her. She knocked on the open door and went in. Gladys's house has three rooms. In the first one, which was used as the best room, there were two armchairs with white embroidered throws over their backs. It was in one of those chairs that Gladys was waiting for death to call. She had been sitting there for more than three years. Every morning was a long wait for the evening. A wait for death. Christine entered the room and sat down in the other chair. She began by

Our Family Traditions and Values . . .

I hope you will observe the traditions and values of our people. We are Kikuyus. Whenever an elderly person asks you to do something you must obey unless you have a very good reason for not doing so. Our practice is that the young always respect and obey the older ones, be they relatives or from outside the family. For example, you should never remain seated while an elder stands. This has to be observed anywhere whether in the home or in public. A young person must always seek permission to talk in presence of elderly people. You're not supposed to joke with people who are not of your age. You are, however, allowed to play and even joke with your grandparents although this doesn't mean you should disobey or disrespect them.

Our clan believes in supporting the needy. You must not turn away a person, especially if their need is for something basic like food or water. Whenever a visitor arrives, you should offer them something to eat or drink. There is a tale that says once somebody refused to attend to a visitor, thinking he was a destitute. It later turned out the stranger in need was an angel. We Kikuyus believe in giving more than receiving.

When it comes to personal matters, for example marriage or sexuality, you should confide with your telling Gladys that she too was HIV-positive, but that she was unwilling to sit down and wait to die. Gladys didn't say much, so Christine talked all the more. She spoke about all of Gladys's children and her own children. Christine said that, between them, they had a responsibility for seventeen children. They simply had to live for as long as possible and never forget that, despite everything, there could always be room for a smile on their faces. They had no right to sit down and wait for death. He would call when the time came, in any case.

Christine kept going back, day after day. I don't know how long she spent trying to persuade Gladys, but the fact is that one day, Gladys left her chair and abandoned her unending wait for night to fall. Christine had succeeded. I asked Gladys what would have happened if Christine hadn't knocked on her door.

"I'd have still been sitting there, waiting to die."

And Christine?

"I knew that Gladys had many children. I heard that she was just sitting there in the darkness. I couldn't bear the thought of that. I thought that I might be able to talk her into making an effort to live longer."

Gladys also said: "I feel infinitely grateful to Christine. But for her, I'd have withered away. When she first came, I didn't want to listen to her. But she wouldn't give up. I thank her for that every morning when I wake up."

*aunt or your uncle. Before making any lifetime
decisions you should seek their approval. Remember,
they want you to excel in life and be someone they
are proud of.*

*Another aspect of Kikuyu tradition dictates that you
should never pass by a person you know without
offering a greeting. Though these days this practice is
falling out of favor it is nonetheless good to know
about it. Those who are contemporaries of your father
should be greeted with the salutation "wanyua" and
they will answer in the same way. Your mother's
contemporaries should be greeted with the words
"wakia maitu" and they will answer with "wakia
awa." In most cases it is the younger person that
should commence the greeting—this encourages
harmony and unity in our community.*

*You must also work hard for your livelihood,
especially because you are a man. There is no
problem that defeats a man "Kirema arume ni
Kigariure," men can find solutions to even the
most difficult problems. The men of our clan
are encouraged to behave at all
times in a reasonable fashion.
Violent conflicts and fighting are
strongly discouraged.*

And Christine?

"I don't think I did anything out of the ordinary. It was just that I couldn't bear to walk past her house knowing that she was there, inside in the darkness, doing nothing, with no will to live. That was all. Nothing else."

· 35 ·

In all I read some thirty memory books while I was in Uganda. Not all of them were complete; some had been interrupted by the death of the author and would never be more than fragments of stories. Some were written by people no longer with us, others had authors who were still alive.

Some were brief, laconic. That could be due to the style or the contents. There were some authors who knew practically nothing about their own ancestors, about the earlier generations of their families. They had left the "my family" pages blank. Other authors seemed to be overwhelmed by the feeling that they had "nothing to say." They thought they led humdrum lives. It had never occurred to them that they would leave any impression behind them apart from the houses they had built, the land they had cultivated, the children they had had. But even if some of the documents were thin, all of them were full of life, and often extremely expressive. Everything in them, whether written, drawn, or pressed in the form of flowers or butterflies—everything was about life and death. Literally.

Most moving, of course, were the memory books written by sick parents of children who were still very small, in many cases infants. They would inherit these slim little books without having any memories whatsoever of the parent who had written this last will and testament bequeathing no money, no property. Nothing but a memory.

There were also memory books written by two parents together. They might not be married, but they have children together. Infidelity is a vague concept in cultures where polygamy has to do with traditions rather than a matter of morality. The infected parents sit together and write these memory books.

These suffering couples. It was as if they were sitting side-by-side, asking: Who are you? Who am I? Who are we? And so their memory books were created.

Needless to say, I also saw unwritten memory books. The pages remained blank. Not because the people concerned had no memories. Not because they had no desire, no intention of writing. They were blank memory books that bore witness to the overwhelming angst that induces paralysis in the face of disease, pain, and death.

These empty memory books were almost always symptomatic of people who didn't dare start to write, as that was tantamount to accepting that death really was close at hand.

It is with AIDS as it is with all other chronic diseases. Many of those infected will refuse to accept that they are sick until the bitter end. It starts much earlier, of course. When many people refuse to undergo tests. Some fall ill and will die with every symptom you can think of. But they insist that they are suffering from something else.

This disease is shameful, burdened with guilt. Whole villages, whole generations are riddled with guilt and shame in the shadow of AIDS. Not everybody is affected in this way, not people like Gladys, Christine, or Moses. But far too many are.

All those who refuse to accept that they are sick believe that they alone will survive. At least, as long as they refuse to start recording their memories in little exercise books made up of a few pages of gray paper.

· 36 ·

One day my stay in Uganda comes to an end. In the evening I drive from Kampala to the airport in Entebbe. There is traffic chaos as usual, with frequent gridlocks: cars, overcrowded buses, trucks with lethally packed loads. The only ones who get to where they want to go are those on bicycles or mopeds, or on foot. It is Saturday evening, the jams are especially chronic. But eventually traffic starts moving again, and we get to the airport in time. The flight departs late at night and I head for Europe, and before long I begin dreaming about people in a coniferous forest.

Their faces are projecting from the tree trunks, frozen faces in wordless horror. The coniferous forest crammed with the dying, and the already dead.

I must be honest. It was a relief to get away. So much death and suffering in a few intensive weeks is more than enough. I shall never forget the people I met. Nor shall I ever cease to be angry over the fact that so much of this suffering is unnecessary.

Christine again: the medication she needed cost twice her monthly wage as a teacher. She earned the equivalent of $55 a month. The drugs, in their simplest form, cost $110. Approximately $1,300 per year. That's $1,300 for Christine, $1,300 for Moses, and another $1,300 for Gladys.

But they shouldn't really need to pay anything at all. When the history of this epidemic is eventually written, a chapter will be devoted to the gigantic pharmaceutical monopolies and the actions of their shareholders and executive boards during the years when AIDS ravaged the world. No courts will be able to bring the owners of those companies to justice.

But the greed and inhumanity tells the story of our age. What we allowed to happen. We will never know how many people died before the drug companies permitted or were forced to permit medicines to be manufactured in places and at prices that made the drugs accessible to the poorest people of the world.

The scale of this crisis is unique. The greed today concerning drug licensing, the ruthless exploitation of the weak economies, the increasing but nevertheless inadequate resources made available to combat AIDS are another scandal. No wonder many Africans believe that the West has no objection to large numbers of poverty-stricken Africans being killed off so as to "ease the burden."

I think about this as I fly to London. It strikes me that these giant airplanes traveling through the night skies are the modern equivalent of sailing ships. In olden days they would ply the seas to Africa at a stately pace.

Nowadays, everything goes much faster. But the distances are no shorter. They are still vast. They are kept vast. They are not distances to be bridged. They are chasms to be left in place. Or patrolled.

The truth about AIDS is of course a general truth about what the world is like today. In other words: what we allow the world to look like.

*I Want to Tell You
How Much I Love You . . .*

*Peter you are my most dear and I love you so much.
Every time I see you I feel like living again. Though
love cannot be bought I leave my bank account to
you and all my savings. Because I love you so much I
want you to take close note of these words: "Keep
away from AIDS." You know this already because you
have seen what this disease has done to others and to
us. But if you appreciate my love, you must obey me
on this matter.*

· 37 ·

It is like one of those awful, cruel fairy tales by Hans Christian Andersen or the Brothers Grimm. It deals with one of the most frequently recurring themes in literature. The possible variations are limitless. Two people, brother and sister, brother and brother, twins, or two people not known to each other at all, are born at the same time. If they are twins, they might become separated only to meet again later without knowing who the other is. As I say, there are endless variations.

Here is one: in November 1989 a good friend of mine, a stage designer, was told that he was HIV-positive. When his male partner underwent tests and was found also to be infected, they were soon able to figure out what had happened. They were frank with each other and with their friends. The stage designer's partner had visited New York in the spring of 1988. He had been careless one night and invited a man he'd met in a bar to his hotel room. There was no other possible source of infection. A one-night stand, death the outcome. Despite the fact that one of them was clearly guilty of making them both carriers of the disease, they never—as far as I know—uttered a single angry word to each other. They both knew the risks. One of them had taken a chance. At that time, in the late 1980s, there were no ARVs. There was no hope at all, in fact. Death would ensue. Soon.

They began to make preparations. Or rather: they decided to live life to the full, to do everything they had planned to do, to cut out everything that was unnecessary. They moved from the town where they lived, settled in the country, and lived a quiet but intense life. I don't know much about their nights and their dawns: they must have been suffused with fear. Then they died, one of them in 1996, the other a year later.

A few years earlier, a friend of mine in Mozambique told me that she had AIDS. Well, she didn't actually tell me at first, but I had started to suspect as much when she suddenly started losing weight, acquired a nasty cough, and lost a lot of her good humor. We knew each other well enough for me to ask her outright: had she tested positive? She confirmed my suspicions. When we went on to talk about it, she admitted that she had started living on borrowed time. She learned for certain that she had the disease in the spring of 1988.

She didn't last long after she told me that she was ill. Although I was able to help her financially, the resources available in Mozambique were inadequate to ease her suffering. Her death was dreadful. Unlike the friends I had in Sweden who were able to die without needless pain, one of them in an ordinary hospital, the other in a hospice.

All three died on the wrong side of the border, as it were. Before this happened, there were virtually no ARVs: afterward, the new medication could give hope to the sufferers. The researchers and doctors had almost reached the first of the finish lines. Only a year or so later it began to be possible, in the West, to slow down the progress of the disease. Nowadays, people with AIDS live comparatively normal lives. A lot end up dying of other illnesses, or simply of old age.

But this development would have made a difference only to my two Swedish friends who died. The ARVs would not have been available to my friend in Mozambique. At least, not unless I had paid for them.

That makes me angry. A desire to overturn the injustice must survive the death of its victims.

· 38 ·

In the early 1990s, at the theater where I work in Maputo, we staged a production of *We Can't Pay? We Won't Pay!*, a play by Dario Fo that has been performed successfully all over the world. In it, a coffin is used to smuggle sacks of flour past a number of watchful police officers. The old carpenter, Mestre Afonse, made the coffin we used from thin plywood. Heaven alone knows where he managed to find this relatively rare but very useful material in Maputo. Anyway, we performed the play many times and then put the production in mothballs as we intended to include it in the repertoire at some future date.

And that is precisely what we did. Two years after the premiere our theater manager, Manuela Soeiro, decided that it was time to give the Fo play another run of about a month. He spoke to me and we arranged times for rehearsals and reallocated one of the parts, since one of the actresses was much too pregnant to manage her part.

The day before we were due to rehearse the scene that involved the coffin I was approached by Alfredo, the stage manager, who asked for a word in private. He was very worried, and stared at his feet. I had great difficulty making out what he was muttering. Then it hit me.

"Are you saying that the coffin has disappeared?"

"Disappeared."

"How is that possible? It was agreed from the word go that this production would have a second run."

Alfredo stammered and mumbled away. I started getting impatient.

"For Christ's sake, that coffin can't simply have disappeared, can it?"

"It has been used."

"Used? What do you mean, used? What for?"

"For a funeral."

I stared at Alfredo for quite a while. Then we sat down in the front row of the stalls. I asked him to tell me the full story. A girl who occasionally used to hang around outside the theater had died. She was seventeen or so and used to beg for food. She had died of AIDS, Alfredo knew that for sure. He also assured me that although the girl probably worked as a prostitute, none of the theater workers had been with her in that capacity.

But it was all about the burial. The girl did not have any relatives. She had run the risk of being tipped into one of the paupers' graves in the city. They were filled once a week with dead bodies. Then the stage technicians at the theater had remembered the coffin that had been used in the Dario Fo play. It might only be a stage prop, a cheap plywood box, but it was better than nothing. So the coffin had been retrieved from the stores and the girl had been buried in a dignified way, though her coffin was only a prop from a play written by an Italian master of farce.

When Alfredo had finished his story, we sat there for ages, neither of us saying a word. I felt sick. It was as if reality had placed its heavy, gnarled hand over the theater.

But the queasiness passed. I told Alfredo that I thought they had done the right thing. No doubt it would be possible to build another coffin.

"Mestre Afonse says he has no more plywood."

"Then he'll have to use something else."

"He has only solid wooden planks."

"Then he'll have to use those."

"They are thick planks. The coffin will be very heavy."

"Then the actors who carry the coffin will have to get used to that."

About a year later, Alfredo and I were both present at a burial service in the big cemetery outside Maputo, by the side of the road leading to Xai-Xai. Afterward, as we were walking towards the gate, Alfredo pointed toward a corner of the cemetery. There were several mounds with no crosses.

I understood without him needing to say anything.

That was where she was buried, in a stage coffin made of plywood which had been used in a theater production.

I've often thought that I ought to write to Dario Fo and tell him this story. I'm sure he would have liked it. I'm certain he would have been moved.

· 39 ·

It is impossible of course not to feel angry about the AIDS epidemic that is ravaging our world. The number of unrecorded cases is astronomical and terrifying. For the majority of those affected, death is inevitable. Only a limited number of those with the disease have access to effective ARVs and the full resources that can more or less control the virus.

The virus can infect anybody at all, anyone who is careless, unaware, or irresponsible. But depending on where you were born or who your parents were, the implications are different. The virus will also infect those who, through poverty, are forced into situations where they are exposed to it. This in itself is enough to arouse and justify anger. This is what our world is like, a twilight zone for poor people in the so-called developing countries. At the same time it is an illusory paradise for those who live in the rich ghettos surrounded by palisades that are growing higher and higher. Death has become an economic question. Solidarity with our fellow men and women is being made more and more difficult.

A growing number of people are forced to accept that their lives are going to be unexpectedly short. They will not be able to watch their children grow up, grow to be in a position to look after themselves. That is why they write their memory books, so that they do not completely disappear from the memories of their children.

In the midst of all this I see Aida and her mango plant. I never saw any trace of her anger, but I am convinced that it exists. Why should her mother have to die when she herself is still so young? Why

*Here Is the Most Important Advice
I Would Like You to Remember
When You Are Grown Up . . .*

*Once two people were in jail and they were given an
opportunity to go outside the cell. When they went
outside one saw gates that were heavily locked while
the other saw the stars in heaven*

*Here are the two basic characters of people—the pes-
simist and the optimist. A pessimistic person will
always see difficulties in every opportunity but an
optimistic person will always see an opportunity in
every difficulty. Believe me in every difficulty there
are both opportunities and problems. It's for you to
make a choice.*

*As I'm writing this I hope you will take note of the
recent work we have done together in raising awareness about HIV/AIDS, me as a sufferer and you as
someone affected. It was not my wish that matters
should turn out this way. I would have liked to see
you grow to maturity and even to have seen my
grandchildren. Probably this will never happen, but
who knows about tomorrow? There might be a cure
for AIDS. I weep as I tell you this. I didn't want you
to hear from the neighborhood that I was an AIDS*

should Aida have to shoulder responsibilities that are much too great for her to bear? She finds herself in a situation in which she has no choice. The only thing she can do is to protest, and she does that by tending her mango plant, watching it live even as she herself is surrounded by death and more death.

This is the point of what I am writing. We must hope that Aida will not need to write a memory book about her own life for her own children. She is aware that the disease exists, she knows how she can avoid catching it, and she will make demands of the man she meets one day.

Memory books are important for Aida's sake.

It will be best if her own is never written.

· 40 ·

What did Aida say when she took me to see the mango plant that she had hidden among the banana trees? Because she was very shy, she didn't say much at all.

I think she felt an affinity with that plant. It was young, as she was. I think she wanted to show that she was able to nurture a piece of life, to make something grow and survive; that she had drawn up her own line of defense, there among the banana trees. Surrounded by death and fear she had planted her little tree as a protection for the living, for things that grow.

sufferer. It's good the way we have handled this issue together.

Work hard, resist evil and you will do fine. I am making arrangements for my sister Mary Wangechi to take care of you in the event of my falling very ill. I don't mean by this that I'll die straight away but death is the destiny of everyone. Treat Wangechi with the respect you have shown to me. Through my experience with this disease I have learned quite a number of things like learning to be self reliant at all times. Copy this. Don't rely on help from others but look after yourself. In case I won't be there continue the fight against AIDS. It's your enemy—remember that it took your mother away. Don't trust people too much. Be cautious in your dealings with them. Associate with others who have undergone what you have undergone. They will be a source of strength. Attached is a list of things I want you to inherit and the contact details of a person who will assist you in my absence.

You're my most loved, the most dear to me. I live because of you. And I don't know how my life would have been without you. You're an inspiration to me and I love you more than I can explain or express.

But I do remember one thing we spoke about. What mangoes taste like. We were in complete agreement: if you eat one mango, you want to eat another one. Mangoes always make you want more. I asked her how long it would be before her plant was big enough to bear fruit. She didn't know, but she promised to write and tell me.

Now, several months after I met her, as I am writing this, I can't help but think about her name. Aida. One letter makes it different from the name of the disease. Just as one hair's breadth separates life and death.

· 41 ·

One night in June 2003, I dream about dead people in a coniferous forest. Everything in the dream is very clear. The smell of moss, the steam rising after autumn rain. Fungi around the roots of the trees, unseen birds taking off from branches that are still shaking. The faces of the dead are inlaid in the tree trunks. It is like wandering through a gallery with an exhibition of unfinished wooden sculptures. Or a studio that has been hurriedly abandoned by the artist.

The faces are contorted. No cries come from their half-open mouths, only silence.

In many ways the dream fills me with unanswered questions. But I know the important thing is that death has a name: AIDS.

If I look carefully enough, at the periphery of the dream, I can see a young and still very fragile mango plant, hidden under layers of twigs that protect it.

And, close by, a half-rotted plywood coffin that once was used on a theater stage but then was spirited out into dark and horrific reality.

We are the ones who decide, nobody else. About what will happen in the trial of strength between the mango plant and the coffin of rotting, black-painted plywood.

Nothing is inevitable.

Nor is anything too late.

The people I have written about here exist in the real world. But their words are not only theirs, the words are also mine. What I have written is a record of what I heard them say and to an equal extent my interpretation of what they didn't say out loud.

In conversations overshadowed all the time by death, silences are often long and full of meaning. I have interpreted what I heard and tried to understand what was not said. I have named some people by name, but the text also contains other people and other stories.

I am full of respect for all the dignity, all the strength I found.

My worry is that not all of us in our part of the world understand that these people need—and have a right to—our solidarity.

H.M.
Sweden, August 2003

Afterword to the North American Edition

Nothing is inevitable.
Nor is anything too late.

"I shall never forget the people I met," writes Henning Mankell after spending "a few intensive weeks" looking at Plan's Memory Book Project in Tororo, Uganda. "Nor shall I ever cease to be angry over the fact that so much of this suffering is unnecessary."

I know that anger well.

It was 2003 when Mankell wrote those words. How would he feel if he were to visit those same villages today?

EVERY WORD INDELIBLE

Henning Mankell is a longtime friend of Plan's. Plan is an international, child-centered develop-

107

ment organization working to improve the lives of children in Uganda and forty-four other developing countries in Africa and around the world. Founded in 1937, we are one of the oldest and largest agencies providing programs in health, education, water and sanitation, and income generation to children and their families in the poorest communities, and a prominent voice for an end to HIV/AIDS.

The idea of writing a memory book comes from a program for terminally ill patients in the United Kingdom. In Uganda it is Plan, through our Ugandan partner agency, the National Community of Women Living with HIV/AIDS (NACWOLA), who began to promote this approach in 1998. The initiative is part of a larger Plan Uganda Succession Planning project.

Succession Planning helps people living with HIV/AIDS to prepare their families for "transition"—meaning the death of the parent and the hard life for children after parents are gone. Since its inception, the Memory Book Project in Uganda has assisted over a thousand parents to pass on their family history this way to their children.

Today, women who once kept their sero-status secret from their closest friends are consulting with their neighbors about the best way to express something, even showing their memory books proudly to strangers—strangers like me.

I have seen many memory books. Like Henning

Mankell, I have watched as infected mothers put all their waning energy into their singular creations, and marvelled at pages made brittle by a loving hand pressing too hard to make her every word indelible.

And the words stay with us.

But the mother is gone.

WHAT WE ALLOWED TO HAPPEN

At the time of Mankell's visit to Uganda, just two years ago, AIDS spelled death for almost everyone infected with HIV in developing countries. In wealthier countries like the United States and Sweden, on the other hand, anti-retroviral (ARV) medications had become more affordable and available to all in need through health insurance or national health plans.

Obviously, ARV therapy is not a cure for AIDS. But the ARVs do effectively stop the virus's attack on the immune system. Less expensive ARVs have effectively changed AIDS from a fatal illness without hope to a chronic one requiring daily care, like diabetes or high blood pressure. Unless you were born in Africa.

In Uganda, ARV medication, when available even as a generic drug, costs about $1 per day. The poor—more than 98 percent of people living with AIDS—can neither find it nor afford it.

While Henning Mankell was with his memory books in the African bush, another HIV/AIDS project was underway in town.

Welcome to the Mukujju Health Clinic in Tororo, a longtime partner of Plan in Uganda. Plan has helped take the Mukujju Clinic into the new century, providing more space and technology to increase the capacity of local communities to provide support services to orphans and vulnerable children in Tororo district.

At the time of Mankell's visit, Plan and Mukujju Health Clinic were piloting a program to stop the transmission of HIV from an infected mother to her baby during childbirth.

Some 700,000 children become infected with HIV each year, almost entirely as the result of transmission from an HIV-infected mother to the infant during pregnancy and childbirth. In Uganda, where AIDS appeared first in 1982, transmission of HIV from mother to child occurs in as many as 25 percent of pregnancies today.

Without treatment, about half of children born with HIV will die before the age of two.

It is hard to ignore odds like that—one in four—but impossible for an organization like Plan. An antiretroviral drug called Nevirapine offered tremendous hope.

One dose of this anti-retroviral drug, given to the HIV-positive mother at the onset of labor and to the infant within 72 hours after delivery, reduces transmission of the AIDS virus by 42 percent.

Until recently, these extraordinary results were only being achieved in urban hospitals serving wealthy patients who could afford the steep prices of ARV drugs. But by December 2003, the cost of the dose of Nevirapine used to prevent mother-to-child transmission of HIV fell to about four dollars, and the Mukujju team began providing Nevirapine to HIV-positive pregnant women, with a single dose to the infant after birth. Thousands of pregnant women have received this lifesaving treatment to protect their babies. Many escaped infection and were born healthy.

However, with the baby's HIV-free birth came the end of treatment with Nevirapine or other lifesaving drugs for the infected mother.

NEXT STEPS

The mothers kept asking us, "What is the point of saving the life of the child when the mother is dying?" Over a very long eighteen months, parents attending the Mukujju Clinic repeatedly asked when ARV treatment would be available to them, so they could live long enough to see their children grow up, to secure their children's future. To extend the life of the parent. To give each child hope.

In response to these parents and to community needs, Plan Uganda has expanded its Mukujju program to include ongoing ARV treatment for infected mothers, thereby becoming one of the first community-based programs in Uganda to provide ARV therapy along with antenatal care, including nutritional supplementation and treatment for opportunistic infections and community outreach.

ARV therapy improves children's lives in two vital ways. For HIV-positive children, it offers hope for a longer, healthier life, very possibly a normal lifespan. For children who are not themselves infected but their mothers are, ARV therapy effectively extends the crucial mother–child relationship. Our commitment is to provide quality ARV medications and continue to do so for the rest of the participants' lives. Plan will move on, but the Mukujju Health Clinic is here to stay.

So, back to my question: How would Henning Mankell feel if he were to visit Tororo, Uganda, again, these two years later?

He would notice remarkably fewer deaths. I think that is foremost. He would see hope in people's faces. Less fear. A renewed vigor. He'd see healthier children attending school, instead of staying home helping the sick.

But he would also find that super low-cost, truly affordable ARV drugs still are not reaching millions who need them. Grimly, some changes take more time, especially in rural villages. And if he stayed awhile in Tororo he could also check in on his Aida, whose mango plant by now ought to be flourishing, bearing delicious fruit.

I encourage you to find out all you can about HIV/AIDS in the developing world, and to do whatever you can to help get ARVs to the poor in rural Africa who will certainly die without them.

—SAMUEL A. WORTHINGTON
CEO, PLAN USA

To learn what you can do to support HIV/AIDS programs in Africa, we encourage you to contact the following organizations:

Hope for African Children Initiative (HACI)
Nairobi, Kenya
hopeforafricanchildren.org
(HACI is comprised of a partnership of the seven organizations which follow—all united in the fight against AIDS.)

CARE
Atlanta, GA
care.org

Network of African People living with HIV/AIDS (NAP+)
Nairobi, Kenya
http://www.gnpplus.net/regions/africa.html

Plan USA
Warwick, RI
planusa.org

Save the Children
Westport, CT
savethechildren.org

Society for Women & AIDS in Africa
Dakar, Senegal
swaainternational.org

World Conference of Religions for Peace
New York, NY
wcrp.org

World Vision International
Monrovia, CA
wvi.org

Information on additional organizations working to fight HIV/AIDS in Africa can be found by contacting InterAction (interaction.org) of Washington, D.C.